RM VAUGHAN

BRIGHT EYED

INSOMNIA AND ITS CULTURES

COACH HOUSE BOOKS, TORONTO

first edition

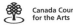 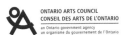

Published with the generous assistance of the Canada Council for the Arts and the Ontario Arts Council. Coach House Books also gratefully acknowledges the support of the Government of Canada through the Canada Book Fund and the Government of Ontario through the Ontario Book Publishing Tax Credit.

LIBRARY AND ARCHIVES CANADA CATALOGUING IN PUBLICATION

Vaughan, R. M. (Richard Murray), 1965-, author
        Bright eyed : insomnia and its cultures / RM Vaughan.

(Exploded views)
Issued in print and electronic formats.
ISBN 978-1-55245-312-4 (pbk.)

    1. Insomnia--Social aspects. 2. Insomnia. 3. Vaughan, R. M. (Richard Murray), 1965-. 4. Insomniacs--Canada--Biography. 5. Authors, Canadian (English)--20th century--Biography. I. Title. II. Series: Exploded views

RC548.V38 2015   616.8'4982   C2014-908413-7

Bright Eyed is available as an ebook: ISBN 978 1 77056 409 1.

Purchase of the print version of this book entitles you to a free digital copy. To claim your ebook of this title, please email sales@chbooks.com with proof of purchase or visit chbooks.com/digital. (Coach House Books reserves the right to terminate the free download offer at any time.)

For my dear friend
and fellow night traveller
Dawn Boyd-Aronson

Sleep.

To dream of sleeping on clean, fresh beds, denotes peace and favor from those whom you love.

To sleep in unnatural resting places, foretells sickness and broken engagements.

To sleep beside a little child, betokens domestic joys and reciprocated love.

To see others sleeping, you will overcome all opposition in your pursuit for woman's favor.

To dream of sleeping with a repulsive person or object, warns you that your love will wane before that of your sweetheart, and you will suffer for your escapades.

For a young woman to dream of sleeping with her lover or some fascinating object, warns her against yielding herself a willing victim to his charms.

– *G. H. Miller,* 10,000 Dreams Interpreted: A Complete Guide to the Meaning of Your Dreams

introduction: Wide Awake

I can't sleep.

If those three words in that sequence constituted a prayer, I would certainly be an earthly saint by now, if not a blessed, white-winged angel, because I say them every night, night after night, and all night long. I've done so since I was ten.

My earliest memories of insomnia come from the long winter nights of the third grade, the deep and deadening black-outs of February in rural New Brunswick in the mid-1970s, an era and geography wherein light or noise pollution would have been purely aspirational on the part of the locals.

There I lay, in my little twin bed, beside my snoring brother, listening to my parents talk in another room, listening to the always-on-but-barely-audible television, listening for ghosts, demons or whatever monsters preoccupied my mind at the time. Listening while my mother brushed her teeth and my father urinated, while my mother puttered about looking for her nightie and my father double-checked all the already-locked doors and windows, while my mother fussed with the thermostat, and, true to his obsessive nature, my father rechecked the locks.

Soon, all was quiet. Horribly, accusingly quiet. Everyone was asleep. What was wrong with me? What, I wondered, was keeping me awake, and was it something I was responsible for? Or was I under a spell, haunted, possessed by the devil? In horror movies and cautionary tales, children who didn't go to sleep met terrible ends, or were snatched in the night, or were themselves malevolent demon seeds.

Midnight would come, and pass, and there I lay, guilty and frightened and angry, wrapping myself tighter and tighter in my blankets, trying to make a cocoon.

I realize now that I was afraid of the dark as a child because I was awake during hours no child should be awake, the hours when small noises echo down hallways and bubbling plumbing sounds like ghostly chatter. I hated the night, hated its stagnancy. I still do.

I am now fifty years old. I have lived in a variety of places, travelled a bit, learned far more than I imagined I would and written several books. I've had a reasonably accomplished adulthood – I stuck to the path of education, followed by a carefully built career and reputation, complete with both clichéd and unusual stumbles. Nothing has changed, however, between me and sleep. We are still at war.

The fact that I have normalized and absorbed my insomnia, adapted myself to its constraints, to the point that I live a relatively productive and stable existence, is indicative of how large the problem is, not of any special talent on my part. It's not hard for an insomniac to live and work and love and play in a world populated by insomniacs. Everyone is sleepy; few of us sleep. The numbers of people reporting sleep difficulties are alarming: 40 per cent of Canadians (Université Laval, 2011), 63 per cent of Brazilians (Instituto Datafolio, 2008), 30.3 per cent of Germans (Robert Koch Institute, 2013), 59.4 per cent of Nigerians (Obafemi Awolowo University, 2013), 40.3 per cent of U.S. residents (National Health and Nutrition Examination Survey, 2008).

Everyone is awake all night every night and, weirdly, many of my fellow sleep dodgers seem to like it that way, and to cultivate a kind of up-all-night bravado, as if sleep is a time waster meant to be conquered. (These would be the same people, of course, who spend hours online watching pets take baths or pride themselves on sitting through an entire season of a cable dramedy in one go – but insomnia, an archetypal blend of keen desire and slapstick frustration, generates irony after irony.) We live in an insomnia culture.

I have watched this culture grow and fortify itself over the decades, as it has played out in my own body and in the cultures that surround me. I've been an insomniac for so long I can't tell if I'm at the vanguard of a new way of living or simply watching a fashionable discontent cycle back to popular prominence. After all, neurological complaints are the Newtonian 'other hand' of technological and social revolutions. According to John F. Kasson, in *Houdini, Tarzan, and the Perfect Man: The White Male Body and the Challenge of Modernity in America*, in the late nineteenth and early twentieth centuries, times of massive industrial and sociological overhaul, neurasthenia, a 'distinctly modern ... disease of nervous weakness and fatigue' believed to be caused by 'excessive brain work ... constant hurry [and] rapid communications,' was the most talked about, and medicalized, social anxiety of the age. The term is now extinct, but the symptoms and alleged causes are remarkably familiar to me.

But it is too easy to suggest that insomnia, and insomnia's cultures, are just the latest unexpected cost of technological advancement, of our Information Age (and thus not a cost so much as a permanent tax, as there is no going back from nonstop connectivity, because that state is too profitable), or that it is merely a faddish preoccupation, the 'new neurasthenia' or the 'new _____' (fill in whatever disorder or disease you last gave money to help cure).

Insomnia is a health issue that has morphed into a cultural condition, like alienation or bullying/being bullied. Insomnia is not just a problem of the body; it's an all-encompassing, polysymptomatic, deeply embedded and perhaps irreversible environmental condition. Insomnia has a culture and has bred new cultures. Insomnia takes a toll on public health, and yet we continue to create environments and attach ourselves to new products and habits that allow insomnia to become more entrenched and more widely experienced.

Insomnia is the enemy sleeper cell (sorry) in the body public – a body about to shut down. The perpetual cycle of hoping for sleep while never getting enough sleep weakens the body and enrages the mind. Insomniacs are grumpy people, as are all disappointed optimists.

Similarly, insomnia culture has created a perpetual cycle of denial and renewal in the arts. I don't subscribe to the notion that creative people are naturally more prone to insomnia. First off, everybody is creative in some way – the 'creative class' of Richard Florida's imagining is a myth that creates a false hierarchy between clever bakers and clever painters – and I have compared notes on sleeplessness with everybody from my barber to my editors. However, insomnia culture, a culture of perpetual restlessness, has a unique side effect on the arts: it creates a default response of endless relativism, of forever looking around, looking for the next bit of stimulus, and thus a reading of contemporary art as being forever up for reassessment and overturning. A painting equals a magazine cover equals a night at the theatre equals an animated GIF of a cat.

As a writer, artist and lifelong insomniac, I know exactly how much insomnia takes from a body and a mind. Some days, I simply can't think. I can't make sentences or complete the simplest projects, but I'm wide awake and easily distracted, indeed craving distraction, as if compensating for my inability to make things by hoarding new information, brighter and faster stimuli. I also know that no two insomniacs experience sleeplessness in the same way, nor exhibit the same symptoms. We are a unique lot, tiresome as that may sound.

So, nowhere in the book am I presuming to speak for other insomniacs, occasional or chronic, and I am certainly not qualified to present any cures, prescriptions or sleep-inducing practices. There are enough people making quack fortunes off Western culture's most persistent, and increasingly dominant, disorder. What follows contains no links to motorized beds, hypnotists, Bane-esque nasal-channel-inflating face masks, pills or herbs or cute behaviourist tricks.

In the following chapters I explore the look and texture of current insomnia culture, and contemplate the long-term socio-economic and cultural consequences of this sacrifice, made in the name of the ever-elusive goal of 'total productivity.'

Over the course of writing this book, I spoke with several sleep experts, my own doctor, another sleep doctor recom-mended to me, the writer and artist Douglas Coupland and many friends. Two distinct patterns of thought emerged from these conversations: first, that widespread sleeplessness is affecting public health because not sleeping has become normalized in our shared ideas of what constitutes 'good health'; and second, that a culture deprived of sleep is not only a less healthy culture, but also one that looks very differ-ent from the culture of even a decade past, because creative people, no matter their field, ultimately make work that mirrors their society.

This book *asks* rather than answers. If the world around us is being run, ordered, financed and even entertained by people who are not sleeping well or not sleeping enough (or, in my case, sleeping barely at all), what kind of culture will we be sharing in the future? More important, is an insomnia culture sustainable? Is insomnia now the new health norma-tive, like extra poundage or blood vessels oversaturated in sodium? And is the wakefulness that surrounds us actually of some value – have beautiful things been made in the wee, twitchy hours?

Insomnia as both a condition and a symptom is a massive topic. People build their entire careers around studying single iterations of the problem. And sleep disorders of other kinds – such as sleepwalking, sleep eating, sleep paralysis, night terrors – are not the focus of this book, as alarming as they are and as much as I feel for their sufferers. This book is my attempt to sort out my own chronic sleep disabilities and, from that highly personal viewpoint (and learned experience), look outward toward a world that increasingly mirrors my lifelong problem, a world that no longer sees the inability to sleep as exceptional, and perhaps even reads *not* sleeping as valuable.

Finally, a note on terminology: the word *insomnia* is an umbrella term for any sleep-disrupting disorder, both chronic and occasional. When employed in this book, the term relates to any medical or psychological situation wherein a symptom is the inability to sleep. Insomnia is both a symptom and a condition that creates symptoms. Subsequently, terms such as *sleep-deprived* or *sleep deprivation* or *sleeplessness* do not refer to enforced sleep deprivation, as might be experienced by abused workers or prisoners, but rather are to be read as events that thrive in a culture that no longer puts value on sleep. For instance, one may be sleep-deprived because one must work late hours. In this case, the term is not exclusively used to describe the imposition of a lack of sleep but also to describe a culture that normalizes and privileges the lack of sleep.

An Old Friend

On forty years in the trenches of the war on sleep

There is an apocryphal Vaughan family story, one told to me whenever my mother brought out one of her over-stuffed photo albums. The story was prompted by a photo-graph, circa 1967, of me, at age two, and a tall man in a white dress shirt and black pants. I think he might also be wearing a tie (I have never been able to find the photo on my own), and he was, to my memory, handsome. The man's name was Reg or Arch or Dave, a short name, and I am standing beside him, wobbly on my toddler legs. He is holding my hand and smiling. My expression is neutral, perhaps bewildered.

The story goes that the smiling man (a family friend, not a relative) used to visit my parents in the evenings for card games and a drink or two – and it was his job to 'walk Ricky' (my name until I turned seventeen) – Ricky, the never-sleepy baby. Family legend has it that sometimes the tall man would have to walk me for an hour or more, because I simply would not exhaust like a normal child, not grow weary after a few rounds of round-the-table. Rocking was no use, warm milk no use, soft music never tried and a thumb daub of rum on the lips only gave me energy.

My mother was eternally grateful to this man, who visited once a week or so and had the patience and energy to walk me in circles until I finally collapsed. I wonder if my mother secretly asked herself if she had married the wrong guy. Maybe it was all a game, a bit of sport. Maybe the tall man was tipsy when he played along. Maybe I was the baby equivalent of a dog that does funny tricks.

Or maybe he was exactly what I was told he was – a nice man. But part of me wonders if, in his kindness, the tall man was actually training me to stay awake, inoculating me against drowsiness. Perhaps I've been trained since I was in diapers to be 'the boy who never sleeps.' I'm certain I liked the attention (I still like attention), and it is possible that my developing brain soon equated defying basic sleep patterns – the baby logic of sleep-at-night – with affection, with being adored and talked about, with sound and light and excitement.

Insomnia has been part of my life ever since childhood; to the point that I thought it was normal. I thought everyone took hours to get to sleep. It's when I made up fantasy worlds to wile away the insomnia. That turned into my lifelong way to deal with it, and therefore I always loved my insomnia, for it was my 'fantasy time.' When I got older and anxiety/depression came to the forefront, insomnia was no longer beloved. Awakening in the night or not being able to get to sleep involved obsessive, horror-filled dread that would amplify with each passing moment. This went on for years until I got a better handle on my depression/anxiety. Which is another story altogether. Now insomnia is back to being my 'fantasy time.'

– D, Montreal

My always-awake teens are a blur. I took some sort of drug every day from the age of thirteen until I was twenty-four. Every day. Pot, speed, acid (lots of acid), tranquilizers, my father's 'nerve' medicine (a wondrous 1970s cocktail of Valium, Syrax and all the early versions of the '-pam family' of antidepressants – my father never met a pill he didn't want to take), Tylenol 3's taken with Wake-Ups, and a cluster of pills I remember only by their colours – blues, reds, oranges.

I also drank the local moonshine – sold by three twenty-something construction workers who lived in a collapsing house by the Catholic graveyard – rum and Coke, rum and orange juice … any brown liquor, basically. But I loved pills. And pills loved me – my ability to stay up after all the other kids had passed out made me a social asset. I could clean up the mess before the parents came home. I could wake everybody who had fallen asleep by the campfire when flashing police lights were spotted rippling over the treetops. I always knew what time it was.

Pills — LSD/acid in particular — heightened my natural (in)abilities, turned what I had considered a curse in childhood into a high school superpower. Drug highs were just another, far less frustrating and far more entertaining version of lying in bed for hours staring at the ceiling: insomnia mixed with a bad case of the church giggles, a twitching wakefulness, but with my own private TV screen in my head.

I was unlike every other stoner teen in that pot did not make me sleepy. Dopey and starving, yes, but never heavy-headed. Nor did alcohol (it still does not). What marijuana did for me as a teen was neutralize the power imbalance between me and my chronic insomnia — if I had to be awake all night, I could at least be amused. And everything is amusing when you're high.

With marijuana, I took control of the long nights and filled my hours with mindless, repetitive tasks, or reading, or staring off into space with the family cat, Taffy, purring on my lap. Being awake until 4 or 5 a.m. was fun, until it suddenly wasn't. Around the age of twenty-three, drugs — marijuana in particular — turned my pre-existing over-alertness into full-blown anxiety and panic attacks, and all the charm went out of getting high.

But I realized through drug use that if I had to be awake when the rest of the world was asleep, I could do something — anything — with the acres of time spread out before me. In university, I became an official 'night person,' a young adult who was happy to set aside the small hours of the morning for writing university papers or cruising the parks for sex (there are always available men at 3 a.m.).

I used to scoff at people who rose at 6 a.m. to work. I, or so I convinced myself, was a more clever person, the kind who used first light for short naps or reading in bed while leisurely drinking a post-late-night cup of sweet tea. Early risers were pathetic people who tried too hard. 'Morning people' lacked sophistication, didn't know what they were missing after 11 p.m. I didn't have a problem, I had a talent.

I never described myself as an insomniac, as an unwell person; rather, I bragged about my inability to sleep. And the academic subculture I immersed myself in not only supported my habits (pulling an 'all-nighter' was almost as worthy of congratulations as getting laid), but rewarded my disorder with a 4.1 grade point average. I was a scholarship darling, on my way to a literally bright (as in never dark, never closed-lidded) future.

As I write the above and read my friend D's account of her own insomnia, it occurs to me that some of the bravado I adopted in my early adulthood to rewire my perception of myself as a person who did not need sleep (as opposed to a person who could not sleep), some of that perverse sense of accomplishment still lingers. It turns up in the oddest situations, like a lie one has told oneself so often it feels swear-in-court true.

A couple of years before starting this book, I decided to try living away from Toronto. After twenty-plus years here, I needed a break. Like many Canadians, I moved to Berlin – one of the world's great night cities. The first year I lived in Berlin, I took great pride in being one of the party gays who didn't arrive at the clubs until after midnight, especially since I was well into my forties. When I have a writing deadline to meet, I get a kick out of sending the finished text at 6 or 7 a.m., so that the editor will see the email time stamp and think I'm a real go-getter (not knowing that I did not rise at 4 a.m. to work, but had never left my desk to sleep the night before). No small part of me enjoys telling people that I am capable of living for weeks at a time on two or three hours of solid sleep per day (I am writing this book, after all).

Ego and insomnia are evil twins – just like other people who suffer from more widely recognized illnesses, insomniacs can, and almost always do, develop a morbid attachment to their insomnia. We like to be asked how poorly, if at all, we have slept. We like our bodies and health to be a topic of discussion, to appear to others as fantastical creatures that can live without the sleep most mammals find absolutely necessary. Our recounting of how few hours we have slept (and we know to the minute how long we have not slept) is the conversational equivalent of showing off a scar, except our how-I-got-this-scar stories can be renewed daily, the hourly count raised or lowered, so we can be offered support and comfort in our distress or congratulations on getting that extra hour of sleep.

Insomniacs develop this backward boastfulness partly as compensation for being so out of sync with the rest of the world, as a way to explain ourselves and our difficulties that does not read as self-pitying, but, in particular after years of suffering, as a kind of lurid attachment. Insomnia becomes our oldest friend, our longest-lasting relationship: a faithful – hellishly faithful – sidekick who we bitch about constantly but cannot imagine living without.

A warty contradiction pops up often in this book, a contradiction I am not certain I can or want to fully resolve. Namely, insomniacs feel alone in the world because they are too often awake while the world around them sleeps. They feel they are both a part of the night and yet singled out by the night's normative behaviours – sleeping and resting. This feeling of isolation is real, as are all feelings, and yet any insomniac can tell you that they also find communities of other insomniacs, and, via the simple revelations of social media, quickly realize they are hardly alone in the world. Why, then, do we feel the opposite? Here we must separate the feeling of isolation from the reality – insomnia creates habits, the most keen and difficult to erase being the habitual feeling, illusory as social media tells us it is, that one is living and enduring a condition on one's one. That sense of being apart from the world is so powerful, it prevents insomniacs from creating deeper 'night networks,' from creating communities of like people. That sounds sulky, like insomniacs prefer to suffer alone and then whine about it later. But insomnia dislocates one from the rest of the world so profoundly that even with abundant evidence that each insomniac is surrounded by fellow travellers, that insomnia is a widely diffused social and health problem, one of the condition's side effects is an inability to step outside of the fraught moments of worry that sleeplessness prompts and create community. Isolation becomes a self-perpetuating symptom.

Insomniacs are self-segregators, which is not the same as being introverted. I have never met an introverted insomniac – quite the opposite. We often appear to be the life of the party – another contradiction. I never used to talk about my insomnia to others, especially not at parties or anyplace fun – but people find out, and they ask, and, if they are solid sleepers, they are absolutely fascinated, as if I were talking about being abducted by aliens. (Actually, I suspect they might be more inclined to believe *that* narrative.)

It would be a lie to say I dislike the attention, and it would also be a lie to write that the 'apartness' that people mark around me does not feed my ego – which all comes back to the horrible but possible idea that insomniacs *learn* insomnia, that at some early point in our development we come to understand that being unwell leads to special treatment, and that we fetishize that situation and, especially if our particularly chronic condition is something that can be replicated over and over for long periods of time (unlike, say, a broken leg), we gain positive reinforcement from being consistently unwell. This dynamic plays out repeatedly until it morphs into a habit and then into an integral part of our personalities.

I have a friend who has several children, all of whom have food problems. Kid One can't have dairy. Kid Two can't have eggs or tomatoes. Kid Three can't eat blue food colouring. The kids keep lists on the fridge of what they can't eat. The lists grow longer every month. From the outside, it looks like a game: Who Can't Eat the Most. And, from the outside, it looks like the children are being taught to not only have bad reactions to foods (at this point, who knows whether or not the reactions are real, feigned, a bit of both or created to please the parents?), but to read their difficulties with various foods as valuable, as something that makes each child unique.

When I was a child, I was convinced that my insomnia was a sign that I was cursed, and I took comfort in the fantasy. Cursed people are special. And so I understand the impulse among insomniacs to indulge in making their sleeplessness a kind of performance, a cocktail topic. It's a way of coping, of normalizing a condition. And, as soon as you mention your trouble sleeping, you will hear all kinds of parallel stories from others. Being up all night can be lonely.

The Stumbling Dead
On the collision of sleeplessness and labour practices

Despite hating leaving my bed in the morning, I will go to great lengths to avoid it at evening time. I get curious about potential TV episodes and other online 'news' late at night. I get creative and intellectually curious and find it hard to switch off and wind down. I get FOMO (fear of missing out) and would gladly stay up till 5 a.m. were it not for the fear of not being able to awaken in time the next morning. It's like I have to bring myself to the point of exhaustion before I can get sleep.

– B, Toronto

In Germany I do see a problem in people always being alert. Smart phones, tablet PCs and other online devices keep us connected and alert throughout the whole day, which is keeping people away from calming down and falling asleep.

– Dr. Med. Samia Little Elk, *Somnologin*, Berlin

While workers today are expected to perform their duties with an unprecedented level of awareness, they are simultaneously being deprived, mostly by the false conceit that less rest = more productivity, of the sleep they need in order to remain alert while at work. The result is twofold: workers now feel they are always at work, at least in their minds, and this ugly but powerful delusion creates a state of hyper-arousal, of perpetual attention.

Familiar refrains: people are less patient today, rudeness is epidemic, attention spans have shrivelled, true conversation is dead, everyone is addicted to technology (at the expense of honest human connection), consumer culture/late capitalism/neo-liberalism won and we are distracting ourselves to death. We don't look anymore, we blink. Our species is devolving.

I am hard-pressed to say any of these popular notions are untrue, but I question the depth of such readings. The problem is not that the human mind is losing its capacity to absorb the complex, or that pensiveness and civility have been replaced by instant gratification and unbridled ego, but exactly the opposite – chronic incivility and a quick-fix, non-stop, live-feed culture are symptoms of our rapidly expanding ability to pay attention to everything all the time.

Of course, it is not nice to go about crashing into people on the sidewalk while typing more observations into your already overstuffed Twitter feed, but let's set aside the moral implications of this now-clichéd behaviour and worry more about how people are able to do so much at once. Sleeplessness is changing how our minds take in new information. And what appears to be rudeness – which is, at heart, a wilful lack of attention to one's environment and co-inhabitants – is actually a new form of social interaction we do not fully comprehend (and thus misread as rudeness) because it is still very much in development. But it would seem we have replaced selective attention-giving with the panoramic view.

A conversation follows a text notification follows ambient noise follows flashing screens follows a ringing phone follows the roar of the crowd. We do this because we have to – the mind deprived of sleep sets itself on high alert, likely as a kind of primitive response to possible danger, danger easily missed when the brain is tired. And thus, cyclically, the more time we spend in this hyper-alert state, the better we get at being multi-focused, and the less we sleep because we cannot (being too alert) and, worse yet, we no longer see the value in sleep. What if you miss something?

Today, we avoid sleep because we believe that time spent asleep is time wasted – but not in the traditional sense, from the post-industrial age, of being time wasted not engaged in labours that directly lead to the accumulation of money, but in a whole new and far more psychologically burdensome sense. Time asleep is time one could use to further develop one's 'essential self' (as the god of the Always Working epoch, Oprah Winfrey, puts it) – time better spent on learning a third language, a foreign cookery or any number of self-improvement schemes, from cardiovascular workouts to mindfulness meditation. The first time I encountered the phrase *lifelong learning* was in the mid-1990s, only a few years after I had finished an arduous graduate degree, and all I could think was: *There's more? More I have to do?*

When work goals and leisure goals (the latter an oxymoronic, but now naturalized, concept) become indistinguishable, the first thing to go is sleep. It is hardly coincidental that compatible (and highly profitable) technologies have arrived in service of the work-leisure fusion. Professional worriers decry 'technology addiction,' but what they describe when they talk about addiction is actually far more nuanced and closer psychologically to mania than dependency, and thus much more resistant to traditional abstinence-based addiction cures. Ever-improving information-sourcing devices are bred from – not the cause of – our current vision of perpetual occupation as success.

The gadgets help us to 'keep up,' but they are not the reason we feel a need to keep up in the first place. A machine cannot dictate what is essentially a moral stance: *I am busy, therefore I am good*. A machine can only reinforce a moral stance, by making the performance of that stance easier, tidier and thus less likely to prompt examination.

Our brains are not being rewired by information technology. Rather, our already problematic relationship with labour (both the paid and the intangibly rewarded) is being smoothed out, made more palatable, by the very devices we have created to do exactly that. If information technology was addictive and therefore as detrimental in the same way as traditional addictions, primarily to our physical health and well-being, there would be a collective movement against it by now, two decades in, as there has been against nicotine, sugar, cocaine and other substances. But movements against devices (which are merely ideologies made concrete), against tools devised to support widely held sets of values, do not coalesce until those values shift. Ask any gun owner.

Furthermore, not sleeping while staying always 'connected' in one's wakefulness has morphed from a puzzling new social phenomenon into an admirable goal in itself – one praised and described with an inverted, morbid braggadocio. Staying up all night, with its connotations of rebellion and Rabelaisian excess (*I'll sleep when I'm dead*), has always had a romantic subtext. And insomnia, when read as a disease, is also loaded with gothic potency, mostly left over from the nineteenth century's investing of ill health with glamour.

But sleeplessness today, partnered as it is with the illusion of ceaseless connectivity (and that illusion's warped portrayal of ambition), is bereft of any pleasurable rock-and-roll energy and/or the moody Goya dreamscape reflectiveness of pulling an all-nighter. Insomniacs are not party people anymore, they are workaholics who take pleasure in both complaining about how tired they are and yet revelling, like high-strung hypochondriacs, in their late-night maladies.

And, unlike previous generations of insomniacs, who spent the twilight hours in solitude (or in small, self-selecting groups of revellers), insomniacs today are never further than a touch away from an entire world of wide-awake, hyper-connected people. We can't sleep, and technology offers us access to everybody else who can't sleep, which in turn creates a backwards race to the health and sanity bottom with the least slept among us the winner-losers.

Again, the technology is not the driving force behind this shared sport (note how conversations among insomniacs often sound like perversions of boasting matches between athletes), but a manufactured commodity sold to accompany (and, inevitably, to also further) a developing need. Put simply, no one has ever been passively kept up all night by a laptop. Because laptops can be turned off. When not sleeping becomes a symbol of one's ambition and also a chronic complaint, a complaint that gives the sufferer so-called bragging rights (another type of ambition), the technology the insomniac is engaged with while awake is irrelevant.

In *Insomnia: A Cultural History,* Eluned Summers-Bremner details how the metaphor of the manic, ever-expanding and ceaselessly chattering 'City That Never Sleeps' – a description formerly applied to New York City that is now universalized – is also an apt parallel with the insomniac mind:

> [C]ities grow endlessly without change of definition; they are instances of 'circumscribed infinity.' The paradox of this built-in illimitability … makes a good working definition of insomnia. Sleeplessness causes thought to feel unstoppable … an effect that increases as the night wears on … And yet the insomniac is equally pressured by circumscription, the agreed-upon time zone when most citizens sleep. Like the city that grows exponentially, creating material blockades – riots, crime and so on – to its idealized infinity, insomnia's mode of increase shortens the night.

Now that entire megalopolises of information, people and virtual structures are available to the insomniac at all hours via simple touch, it is natural to extend the metaphor of the city to its logical and ever-growing conclusion: we all carry sleepless cities around with us, in our pockets and bags, via our vast array of information-delivery devices. We keep the honking, restless metropolis by our beds, can hold any number of twitching spaces in our hands. We no longer inhabit the metaphorical sleepless city, it lives with us, by our side, like a pet. We engulf that fabled space as much as it once engulfed us. The city that never sleeps is inside us.

Throughout the late nineteenth century and well into the twentieth, futurists and speculative fiction creators anticipated a post-millennial world populated by baleful, numbed citizens: people clubbed into passive, heavy-lidded submission by over-bearing governments, forced drugging or dronish labour. The futurists were both right and wrong.

The passivity and apathy that typifies Western citizenship is not the result of mind-numbing, but the opposite. We are too alert, too attentive, too much in the know – and main-taining such high levels of alertness is killing us, while making us much less prone to step outside our particular information streams and ask unruly questions. We are not all turning into zombies; we're turning into hummingbirds – creatures that die if they stop moving. Granted, that does not sound terribly apocalyptic, a Dawn of the Tweety Birds, but just because a thing is shiny and twinkles, it does not mean that thing cannot be lethal. Diamonds cut glass; polished blades slice flesh.

Our attitudes toward sleep have undergone a radical shift. Sleep is held in contempt, read as weakness, something perhaps necessary but not to be overindulged, lest the habit of sleeping for a third of the day dull our ability to do multiple things at once while processing a non-stop stream of information.

The popular idea that our fellow citizens are suffering from a collective bout of attention deficit disorder comes from honest concerns – the concern over possible cultural losses triggered by the erasure of reflection and patience (who has the time to read *Moby-Dick*?), as well as the healthy concern over how we treat each other – but it's not ADD at the root of this massive shift in behaviour, it's attention surplus disorder, a term first coined by the Canadian artist collective FASTWÜRMS. How many things can you do or think about at once? More importantly, how many things do you feel you must do or think about at once?

As a study by the U.S.-based Institute of Medicine put it succinctly, '[T]he fundamental response to sleep loss in healthy people is sleepiness ... In insomniacs, however, it is hyperarousal ... people with the disorder become more vigilant, even though they are sleeping less.'

Jonathan Crary notes in his excellent *24/7: Late Capitalism and the Ends of Sleep* that information and entertainment technologies have always played a part in creating attention surplus disorder:

> Television was only the first of a category of apparatuses with which we are currently surrounded that are most often used out of powerful habitual patterning involving a diffuse attentiveness and a semi-automatism. In this sense, they are part of larger strategies of power in which the aim is not mass-deception, but rather states of neutralization and inactivation, in which one is dispossessed of time. But even within habitual repetitions there remains a thread of hope – a knowingly false hope – that one more click or touch might open onto something to redeem the overwhelming monotony in which one is immersed.

The reward for hyper-arousal and an ever-expanding capacity for multiple levels of attentiveness is the promise of further reward. This is how we are sold the 24/7 false promise, by the possibility of stasis, of finally, after that last click, arriving at that place of complete knowledge and complete satisfaction. The entwining of knowledge and satisfaction is not even questioned anymore: of course one wants to know everything all the time, because with that false satisfaction – never fully realized – comes an equally, and more dangerously, false sense of power. You are what you know, but you don't know what you are anymore, because the self is an atomized entity, a starved fly with hundreds of eyes – seeing everything around it but gaining nothing. The ASD brain does not require nourishment: literal food or the intellectual kind; it requires, and learns to gain pleasure from, if not adore, the *promise* of nourishment, which is really in fullness a promise of stopping, of rest. But it can never rest, because the information does not.

Vigilance plus exhaustion is a perfect formula for both collective and individual impotence. People are not apathetic in the West, as is popularly believed; they're drained. Drained and yet still, always, on the watch.

Restless Leg Syndrome

On my weird neurological disorder, the one that is killing me

My insomnia, like everybody else's, manifests itself in multiple ways. I suffer from a neurological disorder that is under-studied and poorly understood. It's an 'orphan disease,' meaning there are not enough people with the disorder to make further research profitable. It is merely coincidental, but nevertheless usefully symbolic, that the disorder's symptoms include an inability to stop moving – the physical manifestation of attention surplus disorder.

Imagine being tired and ready for bed. You've turned off the lights, brushed your teeth, turned down the blankets and settled your body. Now imagine that just as you are about to lose consciousness, somebody creeps into your bedroom and injects you with an oversized, clown's-prop needle full of adrenalin. Your mind is still foggy, but your physical body is ready to run a marathon. And the adrenalin won't wear off for hours, long after the cramps, the seized muscles and the feeling that your kneecaps are being squeezed between two bricks have dissipated.

My mother once told me that I was a 'kicker' when I was a baby, and that she had to constantly check me to see if I had thrown off my blankets. But don't all children do that? I remember an opposite reaction to childhood sleeplessness – obsessively winding myself tighter and tighter into my bedding.

My first bout of restless leg syndrome – full-on, legs-akimbo RLS – as I understand it now, happened in my mid-thirties, which doctors tell me is typical. It was during a hot summer in Toronto, on a night when I was already wide awake from the suffocating heat. The toes of my right foot would not stop pinching inward toward the sole. The resulting muscle spasms crept up my shin and pumped my calf into a hard ball. This went on all night. The next day, I could barely place my foot on the floor. I wondered if I was having a stroke. My friend Debbie, who was staying in my apartment for a few days and sharing my bed (we always enjoy a good co-snooze, when possible), joked that she figured all that bouncing around in the bed meant I must have been sleep-masturbating.

I went straight to my doctor for a quick fix. He had never heard of such a thing. He tested my reflexes (fine) and heart rate (fine), weighed me (always too fat) and sent me out for a blood test (whose results I never got).

The foot convulsions quickly morphed into flailing legs, and I was kicking Debbie so often her thighs were bruised. She moved to another friend's apartment.

By the time I'd reached a year of doctor consultations and a wide and colourful variety of self-medicating strategies, I resorted to the last refuge of the unwell – the internet. This was 1999, remember. Like everyone else, I still thought the internet was for porn, conspiracy theories and hate groups. Restless leg syndrome appeared after several false starts ('stump and gimp' porn, anyone?). Thrilled, and thinking I'd found a community, I signed up for one of the dozen or so RLS forums, expecting answers and consoling. Typical of any group of people who feel abandoned or overlooked, the forum contributors were a cranky lot, often abusive toward each other and full of wildly contradictory information. Such as the following:

RLS is triggered by salt intake. A salty meal ups the blood pressure and high blood pressure dulls the nerves that signal spasms to the muscles. Drink lots of water. RLS is caused by electrolyte imbalances and over-hydration. Take a warm bath before bed. Take a cold bath before bed. Drink camomile/St. John's wort/evening primrose tea. Camomile contains an enzyme that agitates the tendons in the extremities. St. John's wort is better applied directly to the skin. Evening Primrose causes constipation, which aggravates RLS. Exercise vigorously before bed, or at least take mild exercise, go for a walk. Never, never exercise less than four hours before bedtime. Wash your feet and hands in pepper-mint oil. Not your feet and hands, your temples. Not your temples, your armpits. Avoid red wine. A glass of port before bed settles the body. Watch a lighthearted comedy before bed. All electronic and/or digital communications, passive or transmitting, must cease after 6 p.m. Leave a glowing light on in your bedroom. Sleep behind blackout curtains. Don't eat pork. The smell of bacon induces pleasant childhood memories, like the smell of baking bread. Jumping jacks do the trick. Yoga is the cure. Sleep on a hard mattress, sleep on the floor, sleep with a pillow under your back, sleep with your head hanging off the bed, sleep in a cold room, sleep in a hot room, sleep under heavy blankets but keep your body away from synthetic fibres. Let your pets snuggle with you. Pet dander in the lungs and/or digestive system has been linked to RLS. Take Nyquil, Paxil, Aspirin, Tylenol 3, any of the '-pam' drugs, rub Ben-Gay on your shins. Empty your body with laxatives and purify your system of all foreign chemicals. Do a full lymphatic cleanse. A few bars of chocolate before bed trigger serotonin flares, which override RLS. Read a book. The feng shui experts are right – never have materials containing words near your bed, because words carry thoughts and thoughts carry burdens. Light a candle. No scented candles! Speak to your doctor. The medical industry knows nothing and cares less because there are not enough RLS sufferers to make treatment profitable. All the RLS forums are full of crap. Thank you, RLS forum, you saved my life!

The last time I wandered around an RLS forum, a lively discussion was underway regarding the salt/sodium issue, and whether or not Himalayan salts (the pink kind) are a 'good salt' or a 'bad salt.' One contributor claimed that the lamps made from Himalayan pink salt rocks cured his RLS, another applied a crusty pink jam of monk-sourced salt and organic honey to her legs before bed …

I'm not making fun of my RLS community, such as it is (okay, yes, I am making a bit of fun) – these are desperate people desperately looking for answers to a disorder that nobody fully understands and that the medical world appears to have abandoned. So, of course there are aggravated debates, of course people reach out to pseudo-science and alternative medicine – or outright witchcraft (which is at least more empowering, as the sufferer is given tools and rituals to negate the disorder's power – a seductive and, in my view, wholly acceptable option).

My point is that within the RLS community there is so much division and frantic cure-seeking that people, already sleep-deprived, tend to lose their grip on the real problem. We focus on infighting and our excessive reliance on – indeed fervent devotion to – a singular practice or set of practices, instead of compiling shared experiences toward common cause, or, more important, applying collective pressure on the medical industry.

Any discussion of which came first, insomnia or restless leg syndrome, would not only be chicken-or-egg pointless, but also neglectful of the fact that insomnia is an umbrella term that describes multiple, usually entwined symptoms that feed off each other. There is no such thing as single-symptom insomnia, no insomnia without an underlying cause or subsequent affliction.

An orphan disease, RLS is so alone in the medical family, it is primarily described as a syndrome because no one knows what it really is: a symptom, a disease, a condition ... *Syndrome* seems to be the most successfully vague diagnosis, the one that satisfies doctors, who have to say something, and sufferers, who need a label.

The phrase is awkward, embarrassing to speak out loud. Tell someone you can't sleep because you have restless leg syndrome and the jokes come thick and fast, along the order of 'Me too, but then I just roll the wife over and she takes care of it.' RLS is a diagnosis fit for a *Benny Hill* running (literally) gag, an Adam Sandler set-up line. You can hardly blame the zinger makers. The disease sounds like a pop-and-lock move. I hate saying 'restless leg syndrome' out loud, in full form (but if you just say 'RLS,' you have to explain the acronym, and then it sounds like a joke set-up anyway). Sometimes I shake my legs when I say it, do the joke myself, pre-empt the gag reel.

No two RLS attacks are exactly the same, and no two RLS sufferers display the same reactions, but RLS is generally described, rather uselessly, as the inability during sleep to stop the body from involuntarily stretching, jerking or tightening then loosening (primarily) the leg muscles. If only.

RLS insomniacs will tell you that the leg muscles are only the beginning, a good night. In my own experience, I have bobbed my head up and down in violent jolts, flapped my arms about as if I'd been stung by a hornet, clenched my jaw and the muscles around my chin until my ears rang, laid in bed with my back and shoulders soldier-at-attention style, pinched my butt cheeks together until my sphincter hurt and performed elaborate 'bed calisthenics' (insert your own *Benny Hill* joke here) – rubbing my feet together non-stop for hours, performing stomach-down high kicks, launching a leg, or both, out from under the sheets repeatedly until only my midriff is covered – all while half-awake, during that state of near-sleep when the mind is almost ready to quiet. RLS is sneaky that way – it kicks in only when you are finally settled, finally have your pillows and blankets just right, after the weight of the day begins to lift.

By the end of that terrible RLS-possessed summer, three hours of sleep a night was a winning evening. I was fragile and touchy. I craved cheese and ate it by the pound. I gained thirty pounds in four months. RLS also brought out my latent (but not by much) obsessive-compulsive behaviours – the usual fears and anxieties, the double- and triple-checking of locks, fridge doors, light switches and unclean hands, as well as a quick-thrill/remorse/repeat compulsion to shop daily, to begin idiotic collections of objects (usually holiday- or seasonal-themed), only to dispose of the items a few days later, and, most dangerous, to shoplift. Shoplifting is a crime, but it is also a compulsion, and, as I later learned through talking to doctors, compulsive behaviour is both triggered by and a trigger for insomnia.

Boyfriends came and went during this time as well – nice enough men who always read my inability to snuggle and loll in bed with them as a rejection of either their bodies or of intimacy. When I explained that I was a 'kicker,' they would make that sad face a parent makes at a child they know they have caught telling a whopper. So, off they went, pushed away in all senses.

When your bed becomes the place you go to every night to endure an unstoppable torment, not a place of refuge and quiet, you lose all perspective on the world outside your bedroom because you have no 'safe space.' We are brought up from infancy to appreciate our beds and bedrooms as spaces that provide quiet, rest, solace and pleasure. When that core safe space becomes a site of discontent, physical discomfort, a space one associates with a betrayal by one's own body, you begin to see the world outside your bedroom as being similarly fraught, full of devilish torments and tormentors. So you go online and have a nasty argument about pink salt, because you live in a world where every night you have an argument with your own body. You're trained for combat, and anybody who suggests your latest partial cure for RLS might be less than effective is just looking for a fight.

My First Sleep Clinic
On my search for a cure

I can't remember when I started sleeping badly, but it has definitely increased in severity and frequency with age. 'Sleep hygiene' practices and homeopathy are ineffective, and by now I can mouth the words along with people who tell me what I should be doing to get 'restorative sleep.' Zopiclone works, but then one must decide whether the cure is more damaging than the affliction. Heredity and hormones are the cause for me, I'm convinced. Stresses that are easily managed in the day become malevolent and overwhelming in the quiet darkness. I suspect frolicking hormones contribute to anyone's insomnia, but it's easier for women to connect those dots.

– C, Fredericton

When you are an insomniac or have a sleep-disruption issue, you will inevitably, if you complain to your doctor enough, be sent to a sleep clinic. While each clinic has its own routines and practices, they all do several things in common: basic mental and physical checks, followed by a sleep-monitoring session. You will be told to take a shower and bring clean pyjamas (yes, sleep clinics think people still sleep in pyjamas, two-piece top-and-bottoms sets and nighties, like the kids in *The Brady Bunch*), and electrodes will be applied.

Back in 1999, I walked into the sleep clinic at Toronto's Western General Hospital and was immediately handed a mental illness diagnostic test – the kind that asks you to check off a box if you have ever 'felt that strangers are watching you' or 'heard voices other than your own in your head.' Sleep clinics are not subtle places. After confessing to no interesting mental illnesses, I waited to meet with what I thought would be a sleep doctor. The waiting room was full of warped mirror images of myself: tired people with slumped, worn-out bodies. The desperate, the bedraggled.

The sleep doctor turned out to be a psychiatrist. Psychiatrists are not doctors. They are people who studied medicine but found actual human bodies to be a bit too much work. My contempt for psychiatrists is well earned. I wasted two decades listening to therapeutic advice that ultimately amounted to one phrase: *There's nothing you can do about anything.* And my last shrink sexually abused me (but that's a whole other book – *Troubled*, from 2008). Looking back now, I can almost feel sorry for the sleep doctor who was not really a sleep doctor. How could he know I walked in gunning for his entire profession? But neither of us was at our best that day.

Tall, blond, gym-fit and under thirty-five, the Not Sleep Doctor looked and carried himself like a second-string actor from a police drama, the character who makes the bad jokes in the bullpen and gets killed off in the second season, the loveable-goof type. He put his very shiny brown loafers up on his desk, gave his impressively long legs a lazy stretch and then read my test answers out loud to me, as if I had not just filled them out myself.

The dialogue went something like this:

'So, you can't sleep?'

'I have restless leg syndrome.'

'Let's not get ahead of ourselves.'

'I have all the symptoms.'

'Symptoms are just that. Symptoms. The word comes from the Latin …' (I've blocked this part out of my memory, and wasn't listening closely anyway). 'What do you do for a living?'

'I'm a writer. Sometimes a video artist.'

'I love TIFF! You have your films at that?'

'I make video. The Toronto International Film Festival doesn't accept video art.'

'Oh, yeah? Sounds like a busy life.' He leaned in for the Big Reveal. 'Has it occurred to you that when you go to bed at night you are attempting to replicate your busy day life in your sleep routine?'

I took a long breath and admired his lovely shoes. *I need new shoes*, I thought.

'I'm the writer,' I said, calmly as possible. 'Why don't you leave the cheap metaphors to me?' Remarkably, he did not take the bait. 'What are the treatments available for restless leg syndrome?' I asked.

'Well … there is a medication that has had some efficacy. It was developed for people with Parkinson's disease.'

I believe I actually put my hands together and made a little clapping sound, like a Japanese teenage girl confronted with a new, lime-green animal-shaped purse. Maybe I just did that in my mind. Either way, the emotion was true.

'But it has side effects. Loss of bladder or colorectal control. Spinal-fluid buildup. Headaches. And there is some evidence it contributes to brain tumours.'

'Shit yourself and die.' This I know I said, because I still say it out loud when I bump into furniture.

The Not Sleep Doctor smirked, swung his legs off his desk, clapped his binder closed and bustled me out the door.

'We'll see you next week at the sleep room. Remember to read the instructions.' He smirked.

I remember the sound of his office door closing, a low swoosh followed by two perfectly in-sync clicks.

I never went back.

Fifteen years later, here I remain: chronically under-slept, addicted to clonazepam (which no longer works, but is pure hell to quit), perpetually raccoon-eyed and chubby. The chubby part is likely my own fault, but being an insomniac allows you to combo-plate all your other dis-eases. The RLS comes and goes, usually in one- to two-month-long bouts. I used to think RLS arrived with the change of seasons, or the waxing/waning of the moon, but I know better now – RLS settles in and makes a bad guest of itself whenever it wants. I can have – and enjoy, the way Christians enjoy visits from the Holy Ghost – entire weeks, and sets of weeks, with no quivering or thrashing about apart from maybe a bit of herky-jerky with the feet. These are sweet, treasured days. And then the RLS comes back, somewhat like malaria – without warning or evident triggers.

In many ways, RLS is also a metaphor disease. At the risk of stretching a neurological disorder to worldwide – and thus meaninglessly general – lengths, it strikes me that RLS's unpredictability neatly mirrors the instabilities insomnia creates – psychological, of course, but also economic. An economy built on sleep deprivation rises and falls as reliably, in its frantic way, as the mood swings, energy levels and other ailments of its workers. RLS, the kicking disease, has an appropriately irritable quality, that of a sudden, uncontrollable urge to violence. Furthermore, being both mysterious, in that RLS is neither well understood nor curable, and yet, conversely, systemic (it debilitates the entire body from the locus of the body's prime organ, the brain), RLS is a metaphor disease for insomnia culture itself: a culture fuelled by everything around us, from our work patterns to our habitual distractions, that we nevertheless cannot fully comprehend nor easily root out. Like RLS, insomnia culture feels, at first, like an interruption, a break from normality, then quickly becomes internalized. Once that happens, we kick ourselves awake (to follow RLS-as-metaphor) over and over again until the cycle takes on its own, horribly normal-seeming life. RLS lives in my body and I see it thriving in the social bodies I inhabit. How much longer before the kicking becomes more than a private affair, before an entire society begins to fail and lash out?

Until that revolutionary and perilous moment, I will never stop trying new formulas for sleep. Memory-foam bed inserts, barley-husk pillows, oceans of herbal teas, witchcraft (High John anointing oil, dolloped on polished rocks set on the bedroom windowsill, white sage smudgings, bay leaves with the word *sleep* written on them thirteen times and thrown under the bed), stronger doses of clonazepam, weaker doses. One horrifying yoga class, one stupefying mindful meditation class, head-hammering shots of forty-plus-proof schnapps, 'cleanse' days endured without caffeine, sugar, salt, anything pleasurable ... It's enough to make one wish one had a better understood, systemically treated health problem, like leprosy.

And some nights, I actually fall asleep less than four hours after I've turned off the lights. Some nights, hardly many, and never enough.

If my sleeplessness can't be cured, bigger questions than my own immediate dopey state hover over my body. Will my life be cut short by insomnia? Am I more prone to diabetes, osteoporosis, cancer, inattentive cycling and erectile shutdown? What are the long-term effects on my work, my intellectual capacity (my critics have answered that one, just ask around), the very urge to bother making new things? And now that I am fifty, I can't help but wonder what fifty-five, sixty and beyond will look like – old is one thing, old and haggard is another. Finally, I take no comfort in the obvious fact that I am hardly alone. I am surrounded by insomniacs, both known to me and total strangers. That sleep-hungry look is unmistakable.

Walking After Midnight
On anger and social isolation

My patients come from all classes and are usually between four-teen and eighty years old, average is probably around forty-five. I am focusing on sleep disorders that are of physical causes as well as emotional. Approximately 80 per cent of insomnia cases are caused by emotional problems such as being under too much stress, not feeling safe and comforted at night.
— Dr. Med. Samia Little Elk, *Somnologin*, Berlin

When I first started experiencing long bouts of insomnia, I attempted to cure myself by going for long walks at night. I always chose quiet streets, residential avenues off the main drags. I wanted away from traffic and its busyness metaphors. The impulse to look into softly lit living rooms (from the legal distance of the sidewalk, I should mention), if only for the time it takes to walk past, was impossible to defeat.

Here, I thought, was what happy people were doing, happy people living in happy homes. Healthy homes, where the end of the day was savoured, taken as a reward. Homes where the occupants luxuriated in the pitter-pattering slow rituals before sleep. Homes with lowered light where comfortable clothes and a forgivable slovenliness were indulged, where candles were lit and snacks nibbled … worlds encased in fleece and yellow light, plush caves.

I would walk past these alien domestic scenes and note the details – especially how, night after night, each family performed the same silent pantomime. There stood the tall man in the same grey sweatpants, handing a glass of wine to his wife. There was the local news again, its graphics and camera angles bizarrely frantic. There was the big orange dog on the porch, half-awake, waiting to be told to piss before it came inside, and there was the big orange dog's favourite rug scrunched up behind the front door, matted with fur.

There were never children, not at those hours. There was never music, loud talk, cooking smells or the grind of a washing machine. Not at 11 p.m., not at midnight. It was as if all the sleeping people in the world had agreed to protect each other in the quiet hours, and for many years I enjoyed the illusion of being part of that agreement. I walked like a cat, toes first. I covered my mouth when I coughed. I moved along, unremarkable.

And then I began to hate the sleepers, hate them and their tidy health. While their homes projected gentleness and communal grace to the outside world, I saw only contemptible self-congratulation and moronic conformity. I saw the healthy and rested for what (I thought) they were – false, or at least deluded, unambitious people in quaint, unadventurous homes. People with rules and routines. People I would hate if I ever met. Bores and go-alongers. (As I noted earlier, feeling like the only person on earth still awake while walking past lit windows is one of the absurdities chronic insomnia induces on one's reason.)

By the time my night walks stretched into 3 and 4 a.m., I detested all the comfortable homes sheltering the contented, felt I was surrounded by smug makers and doers, 'quality people' buttressed in their success by rituals I was not party to and had never been invited to learn, only witness. I was outside of the cave – no better, and of no more value, than the skulking raccoons and skunks I met on the sidewalks.

I stopped taking night walks when I caught myself filling my jacket pocket with jagged rocks, the best kind for shattering glass.

Insomnia nags; insomniacs seethe. A potent rage flares and heaves.

Insomnia culture, seeking an antidote to weariness and the misreading of the new under-slept culture as inattentive and 'zombified,' defaults to expressions of rage, the more blunt and aggressive or clever and biting (and rapidly generated) the better, in order to rebrand its fractured, messy, overattentive amorphousness as keen, finely tuned (and attuned), as alert and ready. But, of course, if you are ready for anything, or, more precisely, ready for any number of anythings, all at once all the time, you are not actually a task-solver nor resourceful, you are only ever noticing the tasks at hand, never finishing them: forever biting, never chewing. And that makes you angry. The system feeds itself, fuelled by anger's false energy.

Anger is no longer just a by-product of more deeply felt emotions, as presented in the classical Freudian model, emotions such as fear, isolation or sexual dissociation, a side effect best vented or soothed and subsequently dispelled. Anger has morphed into an ambition, a state of being society rewards, a cultural iteration now industrialized by instant communication systems.

Don't misunderstand me – I am not offering the above from on high. I repeat this cycle daily, sometimes hourly. I take the bait on everything from online newspaper comments sections to social media posts to half-heard, less understood conversations. I always take the damn bait.

When I have gone days into weeks without proper sleep, I eat, drink and shit a kind of touchy but distracted, caustic but unfocused, rage that is misunderstood as crankiness ('having the cramps,' as one friend teases me) but is actually a vocalizing, or text generating, of a vicious and hateful toxicity that I now need and make as much as I do my own blood.

The pattern plays out as follows: I can't sleep; I become angry with my body and mind; I begin my day (which never really stopped); I do dozens of things at once, because doing this tricks me into thinking I am accomplished and thus have defeated my insomnia; then, having to do dozens of things at once, or failing to do so, infuriates me, which feels perfectly natural, indeed like a productive and adjusted response, the only viable response; and then I attempt to end the day while wondering why I am too agitated to sleep. After years of this ritual, I can no longer tell the difference between healthy ambition and spite, or which motivates me to carry on.

And insomnia culture rewards me, and everyone else, for ramping up the cycle. Because being angry all the time at least feels like being productive, because anger-action-response-action-anger exchanges (internal or between me and the world) mimic the progress model of task completion, reward, next-task-anticipation. Maybe that psychiatrist at the sleep clinic, the one who told me I was attempting to live out and sustain my exciting, ego-driven, busy creative life in the off-hours of sleep, was actually onto something, in his tiresomely simple cause-and-effect way.

But how could he have missed that the burning engine sitting across from him, the thwarted fat man with the baggy eyes, was running on waves of spleen and indignation, not narcissism? I would love to be so rested as Narcissus, mythology's most accomplished daydreamer, a man who spends eternity in a daze beside a twinkly pool.

Insomniacs cannot also be true narcissists, because insomniacs are always in contest with themselves. They are, however, often self-deluding. As one fellow insomniac described to me, 'Every night, I have this optimism – tonight is the night I will fall asleep easily … but every night, I am disappointed, of course.' Is this pattern of anticipation followed by failure a nightly reiteration of an already overevolved sense of 'specialness,' a little drama to play out in the dark to remind oneself, again, that one is apart from others, or is this pattern the surface re-enactment of one of the deeper traumas that trigger insomnia: a disappointment with life itself?

As often as we repeat behaviours and thought patterns that make us feel good about ourselves, we do the same mirroring to make us feel bad about ourselves. This is the base idea behind narrative therapy — that we become what we tell ourselves about ourselves, become our own stories. What appears to be the eternal optimism of the insomniac (tonight will be the night!) is actually the opening act, the false 'everything looks fine here' set-up of a well-rehearsed and thoroughly memorized play, a play that ends, like a backwards bedroom farce, with all the players in bed doing nothing but waiting.

My friend described her nightly game of hoping against hope as an act of optimism, but how can anyone be optimistic for so very long and so very many times? It is more likely that that performance of optimism is a survival prompt, something akin to whistling one's way into a darkened room, the plot device in the nightly drama that gets her down the hall to the bedroom, where the real story begins, again.

The insomniac's anger is unique and ugly. Insomniacs blame themselves for their inability to sleep, and the well-slept agree (we are told that our habits, even our body sizes, are at the root of our misalignment with the day-to-night world). Insomniacs create patterns of self-loathing unimaginable to the rested classes. And every negative impulse or action an insomniac performs she automatically traces back to her inability to sleep, because that inability becomes part of how she identifies in and against the larger world.

Insomniacs accept all (and any) blame much in the same way they will also try any cure, and from that blame, patterns of behaviour form, and are gradually attuned, that separate the insomniac from others. We are uniformly difficult to manage, and our motives are mysterious. We are mirrors of our condition. We delight in narratives that affirm our apartness, revel in conspiracies and half-truths, and distrust the essentials of person-to-person communication — words, tones, facial expressions, body language.

Deprived of the primal shared experience of rest, we grow isolated. Humans are inherently social, sharers of the same cave, except for those of us who sit outside the cave walls shaking our heads at the night sky.

> But illness a form of depravity? That is to say, not originating in depravity, but itself depravity? That seems to me a paradox.
> – Thomas Mann, *The Magic Mountain*

Why won't my mind settle, go quiet? Do insomniacs suffer from sleeplessness or indulge in it? Is insomnia a type of mania? These are perhaps metaphysical questions, so let's pursue them along those lines.

What is insomnia, truly? The inability to let go of one's immediate reality, or the opposite: a heightened – to the point of near dissociation – awareness of one's present reality. And I do not use the word *dissociation* lightly.

I've imagined all sorts of utterly unreal, or all too real in the moment, things in the middle of the night, things that go bump or that I wished would. Insomniacs are often as prideful as they are beleaguered. We count the hours we do not sleep until they become a perverse collection, because self-indulgence is the insomniac's best and worst habit. If we can't be like normal people, we want to be the *most* not-normal. Pride is an unconquerable human need, even in suffering.

When I talk to other insomniacs, games of 'sleepless poker' quickly begin. I only got two hours last night, I will say, for instance, and that will be countered with 'two hours, two whole hours?' And the game begins, the race to the metaphorical bottom, the sweaty, tangled sheets at the foot of the bed. All insomniacs do this; few admit it.

What if I was cured tomorrow? Would I miss my long identification as an insomniac? And does that identification through illness, the sense of the self as less-than, constitute a form of depravity, of wilful misalignment with the world of health and stability?

In Thomas Mann's novel *The Magic Mountain*, a group of abject neurotics meet at a mountaintop sanatorium and slowly die in front of each other over a period of several long and very chatty months. They are all dying from consumption, but the cause hardly matters. What consumes them is their relentless need to categorize and sub-categorize, enact and re-enact. Each patient wants to be the least healthy, the most ruined and yet also, and this is key, the most informed. The patients, ranging from a young man in his prime to a clearly psychotic elderly woman, each lay claim to being the greatest and, again, this is key, the most obvious sufferer.

Conversations in the novel, long and winding conversations that appear to be about anything but illness, are always exactly about illness, only disguised. Mann's novel is a horror show where all wounds are ultimately self-inflicted and, most disturbing, thoroughly beloved.

I read *The Magic Mountain* while writing this book. Perhaps not the smartest idea, but the mind goes where it wants to go. I identified with every single character in the novel, in the sense that I too cross the proverbial thin line between love and hate with my disorder, that I too live in the paradox of engaging my illness as a form of subjugation – in that I endure my sleeplessness as a victim and pay for it daily in ill health – while engaging with, monitoring and tending to my sleeplessness as a kind of practice, a performance. Insomnia defines me as much as defies me, and its lifelong presence has become one of the few reliable facets of my existence.

This 'relationship' between me and my disorder warps everything I do and make. The idea that the unwell take a reversed pride in their illness is hardly new or novel. But were I engaged in daily familiarity with anything else as destructive (to myself, to the things I make, say or do), and as against nature itself (and simply dismissing 'nature' as a construct, like 'gender' or 'normality' has lost its charm for me), surely this ongoing fascination would be marked as a depraved action, one both outside of common sense and wildly mono-maniacal. And then to make art about it … that is a hall of smeared mirrors.

I acknowledge that my insomnia is both real and constructed, a product of both lack and reward. Actual not-sleeping is only the start. Perhaps it was always ever only the start. Perhaps I have built my own dreamless empire.

I'm a writer and an artist, so it would be silly not to talk about the long-standing connection between creativity and insomnia – or, rather, the alleged connection. I know many artists of all stripes who have difficulty sleeping. I also know several academics, one IT manager, an accountant and a dentist who suffer from insomnia. And I know many artists who put their heads to the pillow and are out for a solid eight hours, every night. The romantic idea of the sleepless artist is not only a cliché, it's a useful tool for people who profit off creativity to employ indirectly when workers complain about lack of rest. *You're creative, you're supposed to be up all night clutching your skull, tortured by doubts.* No. No, we are not. And this is not the nineteenth century. Goethe is dead.

There are studies that attempt to link insomnia to high levels of creativity (the idea of ranking creativity is obnoxious to me, but that's a side issue), but they are based on what appear to be carefully selected anecdotes. One questions their value, or purpose, given that we now live in a 'creative economy' – to me, they smell of an indirect attempt to justify a health problem with inexact, old-fashioned ideas of both what constitutes creativity and what fuels creativity.

Nevertheless, the evolution of an insomnia culture must also include the evolution of insomnia cultural products – works made within the context of a sleepless era, not necessarily by insomniacs nor actually about insomnia itself, but from the larger context of a culture that no longer makes or cannot make time for sleep. I focus here on the visual arts and performance art, the fields I work in myself. There are parallels in all the arts, of course, but these are the disciplines with which I have the most experience.

Every decade or so, someone with a lecture tour to sell or a book to hawk declares that Art is dead or that Art has a whole new meaning, or needs to have a whole new meaning. The most recent case is Alain de Botton's book *Art as Therapy*, a kind of pop-psychology guide teaching the reader how to look at art as a personal self-improvement tool. Art, however, never changes, it just moves around, shuffles the pieces on the chessboard. But the dream of a return to an old-fashioned way of reading art, one that will heal wounds, is perhaps too tempting for de Botton's followers to pass up. However, now that insomnia culture is the default pop culture, art can't be relied on at all – because our sleep-starved minds seek the impossible: reassurances and comfort simultaneously presented with abject distrust of the concrete. We don't sleep, and so we don't dream, and when we lift our heads off our desks to make new things, be they loaves of bread or epic poems, we no longer understand what fuels our creativity. It's a testament to our stubbornness as a species that we continue to make things at all – unless we account for the seduction of submission.

The tired mind seeks comfort: in the familiar, the easily parsed and the childish (as in reminiscent of childhood amusements, although a babyish tantrum would hardly be out of order on occasion). The insomniac mind – individual and collective – is defined by resignation, both morbid and casual. If you have not slept properly in days, you stop trying to figure things out and come to the grudging conclusion that most questions are not worth the intellectual energy. You avoid the dialectical, points and counterpoints, and lift your shoulders in a 'whatever' gesture. In the case of the arts, you shrug off whatever has the potential to either confront or be didactic. The insomniac mind is beyond being too tired to sort out issues; it shuts off the intellectual urge to problem-solve, and seeks comfort in a low-grade, profoundly (and chicly) disinterested, reflex nihilism.

Worse still, when one takes life cues from one's experience of 'culture' and the arts, and applies this shrugging resignation to any curative formula for sleeplessness, one creates a perpetual cycle of reading everything put in front of you as just one more rivulet in an ever-bubbling stream of related but ultimately unsynchronized information. Nothing works or matters, but everything is worth observing.

Contrary to popular opinion, and the simple logic that less sleep = less creativity or less imagination, contemporary culture is marked not by lack – neither a lack of talent or commitment on the part of its makers – but by aversion. To talk about contemporary culture as a by-product of insomnia is not to describe cultural products as failing in traditional categories used to assess works of art, because insomnia culture allows participants to wilfully avoid what we traditionally describe as the 'basics' of any genre: insomnia culture thrives on nebulousness and a blurring of boundaries. But this is hardly because its practitioners are incapable of creating the so-called skeleton, any given genre's infrastructure; it's because those infrastructures do not suit insomnia culture's purposes. You have to know the rules in order to break them, after all. Or, to be more precise, to realize the rules have no value to your project.

Because the insomniac mind favours mild amusement over strenuous investigation, dream logic over stratagems, insomnia culture's products typically avoid the traditional lures of entertainment – narrative through lines, vivid characterization and reliable structures, problem-situating and/or problem-solving, arguments and positions, the affirmative in general. What they don't provide in 'hard' story-building, products of insomnia culture more than amply supplement with buckets of whimsy, random anecdote and flashes of urban near-surrealism.

An insomnia culture artwork will never share a revelation with an audience; but the audience, already strained by attempting to keep up with the well-slept world, does not want questions answered or puzzles solved (or even presented) anyway — it wants cute animals and gentle lullaby melodies, sweet faces and velveteen textures, microscopic observations. In the context of literature, such works have been described by critic Jonathon Sturgeon (and others) as 'autofictions,' 'a new class of memoiristic, autobiographical, and metafictional novels ... [wherein] the life of the author is now the novel's organizing principle,' because they rely heavily on the promise, or premise, of fiction, of a made-up world, but are actually recordings of events as they transpired in front of the author, gentle and often genteel acts of record-keeping.

In the visual arts, insomnia culture has created two distinct streams — the infantile and the absent. Several years ago, I attended a hybrid performance and visual art event conceived and played out, live onstage, by a prominent Canadian artist. I loved it. The audience was comprised mostly of millennials, plus the usual art-world crowd and, strangely, a stern group of visiting artists from northern Europe. After the event, which featured toy-instrument music and drawings of woodland creatures, one of the clenched-face Europeans turned to me in disgust and asked, 'Why do so many Canadian artists make art for children?'

It was true that I had at that point seen an inordinate amount of art that could politely be called faux outsider and impolitely labelled twee. My reading of such works at the time, one I wrote about in various publications, was that young contemporary artists were sourcing their imagery, style and discordant presentation strategies from the outsider, or raw, art movement — i.e., from works made and intentionally positioned (and marketed) as having come from disenfranchised and unschooled communities, such as self-taught folk artists and the intellectually challenged/differently abled/mentally ill. At the time, I dismissed this phenomenon as a pose, a clever but empty style choice, made by the informed who were actively poaching from the uninformed, the less lucky.

Now, almost a decade later, I see this emphasis on the cute and homespun, the lyrical but never lyrically complicated, for what it is – the result of a generation of artists growing up in an insomnia-driven culture that neither wants nor can possibly, except on their best and rested days, process cultural products that do not mimic their idealized, and much sought after, version of a soft, fluffy dream state. And what else could that dream state look like but an insomniac culture's last full memory of dreams – the sleeping visions of big-eyed animals, soft nursery colours and twinkling sounds?

Furthermore, since that cultural moment, insomnia culture's cultivated infantilism has permeated into advertising, graphic art, home décor, fashion, music videos, restaurant menus ... the entire pictorial realm. You know the look – dynamic but intentionally flawed, with imprecise lettering designed to look handcrafted by an eighth-grader, Crayola tones, pictures (hand-drawn or made to look hand-drawn or skilfully photoshopped to mimic a beginner's pixel-scratched understanding of photoshopping) of animals, crypto-zoological creatures, plus human characters derived from storybook archetypes, such as the mustachioed villain, the fairy, the manly woodsman. Despite all immediate evidence to the contrary – i.e., the supposed lack of polish, a keen meme-readiness – insomnia culture art is very well informed about its place in the faux-outsider-imagery stock exchange.

A simple way to test the prevalence (and commercial power) of insomnia culture's visual turn to the infantile is to visit a stationery store. Stationery follows trends and the public mood, and then quickly copies what it discovers, faster than any other mass-generated product, because stationery is inherently disposable, meant to be bought and sent out again. On the greeting-card racks you will see many examples of carefully 'raw' renderings of beloved animals. The animals may change – last year it was stags, this year it is foxes – but the look remains babyish, soft and sweet. Their messages can be summed up as variations on a nodding, post-ironic (and deeply uninvested) pat-on-the-back 'Everything is okay,' conveyed graphically in a manner that reminds the viewer of pencilled love notes sent between high school students, and matte, slightly rough, card stock, paper that triggers tactile memories of woolly blankets and crib textiles.

At this point a personal disclaimer is necessary: I consume plenty of the products described above. Arguably, the cover design of this book falls under the same category. I have never had a problem with cuteness, because there has never been a shortage of cute's opposite, brutalism, in my world. So, while I recognize this visual style as a by-product of insomnia culture's dulling of the senses, I am not condemning the consumer taste for the faux outsider. Happy is as happy looks, or sells.

On the other hand, it is hard to love the high-end, viewer-excluding cousin to the faux outsider, insomnia culture's elitist fascination with New Minimalism. A hybrid of 1970s grey, scarcely present Minimalism and digital imaging (but often digital imaging manipulated to look analogue), the New Minimalism, in its preoccupation with blankness and sensory negation, perfectly encapsulates insomnia culture's innate rage, a rage borne of hours of staring up at the dead landscape of the bedroom ceiling.

Minimalism has always contained a reactionary element – mostly against the equally reactionary decorative, kinetic and populist art movements. The New Minimalism, however, lacks any political or socio-artistic agenda, despite its abundant use of worn cultural theory as an explanatory crutch. New Minimalism is simply a reflection of insomnia culture's practical, real-world side: when you live without consistent sleep, you spend a lot of time in darkened rooms, colourless worlds made up of blacks and greys. Unlike the first iterations of Minimalism in the 1960s, borne of a growing distaste for the decorative, which was considered conservative and bourgeois, New Minimalism has no political or social agenda, no desire to alter a collective consciousness. It reflects more than it shines.

New Minimalist artists desperately comb their underwhelmed senses for any sign of life, and allegedly find beauty in pathos-inducing objects such as mass-produced light fixtures, fluorescent tubing, 'neutral' domestic appliance colour schemes and scanned-then-rescanned-to-near-erasure photography. New Minimalists, much like children who see monsters in their closets, see elegance and even glamour in objects that, taken out of the sham rarefied air of the white cube, would barely attract attention if left in the middle of a busy highway.

New Minimalism is insomnia culture's waving of the (bleached) white flag of surrender. Sleep deprivation creates a state of mind wherein the abject unimportance and utter lack of visual information of, say, a strip of cladding, a concrete block or an artificially negated photograph, becomes loaded with romantic resonance: the banal made bountiful. As they might in a dream state, if they ever got there, New Minimalists invest the ordinary with latent powers, systems of meaning and symbolism that said objects never owned in the first place or were ever devised to project – all of which would be fascinating, on a psychological level, as a kind of shared act of mass dissociation, if the final product, the actual works on view for the viewer, were not so deadening and easily shrugged off.

A curious note on New Minimalism: I have yet to see a New Minimalist exhibition that took more than forty-five seconds to fully regard and, sadder still, fully comprehend – which is a sad irony, given that the insomnia-ravaged mind always has time to kill, hour after late-night hour.

Also, visit any three exhibitions from the school and you'll notice that at least two of the shows use mirrors, especially mirrors positioned to create a distorting and/or disorienting effect. While this may seem dissonant and not in keeping with New Minimalism's distaste for showmanship, it is actually the genre showing its hand, revealing that underneath the 'So what?' absenteeism lies a cluster of conflicted emotions, primarily those relating to self-image.

Insomnia culture is nothing if not self-loathing. We can't sleep, we tell ourselves, because there is something wrong with us, with our bodies and minds. We are being betrayed by our own neurology. We must not be deserving of rest. This constant state of war with the body breeds a melancholy narcissism – nobody understands our special condition, our apartness from the well-rested world. The mirrors and mirror play so common to New Minimalist works is a concretization of this negative narcissism, a literal reflecting pool, affirming our feeling of apartness while reinforcing our very real sense of just how bedraggled we look. It is also an aggressive challenge to the works' visitors – see yourself as I see myself, nightly.

In the endless loop of reflection/object/re-reflection, a simmering hatred for the healthy world boils. Mirror play is the tipoff – the 'tell' – of New Minimalism's jealous glare. New Minimalists ask us to find beauty in paper clips, doorknobs, typography treated as religious relics, found scraps of metal or washed-out, distressed images (to name but a very few exhibition centrepieces I have witnessed) because insomnia culture creates contradictory impulses around the banal. The paper clip that resonates at 2 a.m. becomes just a paper clip at 2 p.m., and the resultant exhibition takes on the form of a dare, one directed at any viewer who questions how the paper clip got to the gallery floor in the first place.

I've zeroed in on the visual arts in my depiction of insomnia culture's commodities because it is the field in which I make my money, as a commentator and occasional contributor, via video and performance – and yes, I too have my faux-outsider, abject moments: a recent video project created in Berlin involved me standing in front of various famous local landmarks, dressed sloppily in dark jeans and a bland grey T-shirt while sporting a dead-inside, blank look, and then falling down, over and over, turning my entire body into a slumped expression of disconnectedness.

Insomniac culture, drained of the ability to enjoy visual art that does not come with disclaimers (presented up front or obviously implied), a handicap bred by the subliminal fear that one has actually, finally fallen asleep, but at the wrong time and place, demands that all visual signifiers nod and wink, hard and often, to their consumers and reassure them that, yes, what is before your eyes is not meant, not a presentation of a set of ideas, but rather a presentation *about* presentation, a layering of visual codes driven primarily by its own clever positioning(s) and not any outdated ideas of transportation, or base pleasure-giving. Insomnia culture's perverse puritan streak (again, a product of insomnia rage) is never far underneath, with 'realness' standing in for wholesomeness.

To wit, a perennial favourite of insomnia performance art is the 'performed lecture.' One sits down and is told that the people onstage are whoever they are in real life. The stage resembles a classroom or simply contains a podium (there is almost always a chalkboard as well, or a digital projection that illustrates the subject at hand). Music, costume, makeup – any of the delicious artificialities of theatre – are wholly absent. The performer/lecturer walks onstage, speaks to the audience about a subject, usually of some topical socio-economic or environmental nature, and then ends the lecture. No one present has been 'fooled' into believing the person onstage was representing, enacting or pretending to be another. The stage is nothing but a platform for the delivery of information – a live version of a laptop screen stripped to the bare essentials.

Insomnia culture's terror of creating imagined or constructed spaces, spaces that might mimic (or be informed by) the dream state, a state insomniac culture has made so deeply alienating as to be read as a threat to the authentic, neuters both the performative impulse and its tools. Acting is silly and artificial, scripts are lies, a decorated stage is an insult to a truly informed audience (who cannot take pleasure in well-crafted artifice to begin with, because the sleep-deprived already have enough reality/not-reality challenges). That insomnia performance art is almost always a crushing bore goes without saying. It is meant to be good for us, like New Minimalism.

Insomnia culture makes us perversely comfortable only when we feel profoundly cheated, or, more perverse, when we are let in on the cheat from the beginning.

Counterpoint
On chatting with power sleepers

I've had much more trouble with it in the past, until my doctor told me to take Benadryl each night. It still hits me if I've eaten too much too late (Oh! for the stomach of yesteryear), slept too well the night before, am excited about something good or am upset about something bad.

– F, Atlanta

I can never get enough sleep. I never suffer from insomnia.

– A, Toronto

The three M's: melatonin, masturbation and marijuana.

– T, Toronto

I rarely have problems falling to sleep and sometimes envy people who are able to live a longer (and just maybe more productive) day than I am.

– P, Toronto

I'm a fan of Canadian author and artist Douglas Coupland. I've written about his work several times and I've had the pleasure of meeting him at various events over the years. He is, despite his celebrity, approachable and charmingly self-effacing. And completely in disagreement with my ideas around insomnia and the culture of sleeplessness.

While writing this book, I encountered an online interview with Coupland wherein he mentioned that he often sleeps half the day. I was both jealous and curious. Coupland's novels (*Jpod* and *Microserfs* come to mind) often function as how-to books for managing your life, or mismanaging your life, in the information age. Although, as you'll see below, he is not entirely on-board with the popular perception that technological advances in information-sharing are changing how our brains function, if not our innate humanness – nor am I, but mostly because I am not a neurologist and will leave that Big Question to scientists.

Reading that interview, I decided to interview Coupland myself, via email. I was hoping for some wise thoughts on what is happening to sleep – not for simple 'blame technology' affirmations, but insights into my own research and experiences. Through a mutual friend, we connected and, to my initial horror – and now, on second glance, delight – Coupland could not have agreed with me less. Here is the transcript of our email exchange.

RM VAUGHAN: How is the push-pull between constant awareness – 'tethering' by technology, if you will – and need for sleep, now described as 'the new fat' in health circles, changing the way our minds function, especially the creative part of our minds?

DOUGLAS COUPLAND: So many ideas embodied in one question – but I don't agree with its underlying assumptions so I don't think I can answer it. Sleep is sleep. It goes back hundreds of millions of years, and can't be so instantly obsolesced by something new and blippy like online life.

RMV: I am arguing that we have now naturalized lack of sleep to the point that we have created an insomnia culture, complete with its own art forms and styles. Responses?

DC: I have to totally disagree. I think insomniacs are insomniacs by nature – and that's how they're built. Worrying about lack of sleep is far more stressful than actually losing sleep – or thinking you've 'lost' lost sleep – as if the sleep you could have had went off to some cosmic dumpster. Just because you maybe slept more when you were younger doesn't mean you need it when you're older. The most vibrant people I know get four hours of sleep a night. They embrace it and it seems to work.

RMV: Why is there so much bravado around not sleeping, where does the romance of staying up all night come from and why is it still a powerful cultural cliché (in everything from pop songs to YA vampire fiction)?

DC: Everyone stays up late when they're young ... unless you're like my brother, who has woken up at 6 a.m. from kindergarten onward. But yes, people sleep much less as they age.

RMV: You said that you sometimes sleep for twelve hours, but when you do get insomnia, it drives you crazy. What do you do to cure it?

DC: Sure, but it always goes away. I love sleep and build my life around ensuring I never have to wake up to any sort of obligation ... which is why all my meaningful meetings or what have you take place after 2 p.m. Pacific time. If I get insomnia I know it will pass. It could have been caused by so many things ... something I ate on a plane; a TV show that tapped into my deeper self; generic stress. Again, I think the worrying is much worse for you than the actual sleep loss.

RMV: If we are entering a period wherein people sleep less as a career-enhancing choice or to comply with fashions, what will the resulting culture look like?

DC: Hmmm ... I just don't agree with this. I'm sorry ... but I just don't. This is so grim and despairing. Sounds like you're having sleep issues across a long span of time. Is it the lack of sleep or the worry about that lack that troubles you?

RMV: Why do we blame technology for our sleeplessness (as do pop doctors and the like), but at the same time want more and more of it? In other words, why are we always in a love-hate relationship with information-delivery machines?

DC: I don't understand this question. Sorry ... I just don't get it. I really don't.

RMV: Finally, how do you think your own sleep patterns affect your creativity?

DC: I can only speak for myself. Say I foolishly plan a noon lunch in downtown Vancouver. That means I have to be in the car by 11:15 a.m., which means I have to be up by 10:15 a.m., which means that from 6 a.m. onward, I wake up every eleven minutes wondering if it's 10:15 yet. Which is a total fucking disaster, which ruins all creativity for the day, and whatever the lunch was, I sit there hating you for ruining my sleep. If I book lunch with you, it means you cost me $1,000 minimum for a day's lost creativity with a resentment surcharge. I hate this so much that I don't care who you are or how worthy your lunch is. Fuck you: no lunch. I think I'm not alone on this. Creative nighthawks trying to have a normal persons' lunch is just a waste of human spirit.

I don't think I was much help to you at all. Sorry. But my sleep experience is the opposite of most people's.

This exchange has to go down as one of my best/worst failed interviews, right up there with my conversation with film actor Carrie-Anne Moss, who answered every one of my questions for the *Globe and Mail* with one word: No.

I have a number of takes on this exchange. First, that my questions were confused and confusing. I was nervous as a kitten corresponding with Coupland, and I'm not certain why.

Movie stars don't scare me, and in my previous job as a celebrity botherer for the *Globe and Mail*, I met some real live monsters. Likewise, artists never unnerve me (they are mostly glad for the press), but Coupland ... he's just so damned confident and accomplished. Take one: I blew the interview.

Take two: he's right. What's the big deal about sleep? Sleep is as mammal-normal as shitting. Coupland has no trouble. What's *my* problem?

Take three (I'll call this the compromise position): people who have no trouble sleeping will never understand what it is like to live year after year with a sleep disorder, and, also, to someone whose entire art practice has been arguably an extended examination of technology culture(s), my questions were simple-minded. I'm resigned to the disappointment of the latter.

Why, then, include this exchange at all? First off, for transparency: second, because only interviewing people who agree with me would be less than entertaining, and I find this entire transaction abjectly funny, a kick to my own pants; and third, because, in the back of my mind, a part of me agrees with Coupland.

After all, Coupland is one of the most prolific and successful artists of his generation. He's a brand now. And he obviously has a handle on the sleep-to-work ratio. How much of my own sense of my creativity is both bound up by thinking that I do less because I sleep less and, conversely, that my insomnia is part and parcel of my creativity, that I am an insomniac because I have a brain that will not stop foraging for and reiterating new information, a brain that never 'quits'?

Coupland's merciless tone does not offend me. I will always blame myself for my inability to sleep, always think of it as a personal failure, not as a convenient and shame-free extension of a much larger cultural shift or malaise. I see how Coupland's answers mirror my own deeply entrenched self-blaming, and

I am not writing that to solicit pity, but to point out the bald truth that every insomniac knows: it is always your own fault. Even when you are enraged by the sense that you are being judged, or feel that you've been labelled a person making a mountain out of a sweaty pillow, another part of you says, 'He's right, get over it, and sleep is not so important anyway.'

In many ways, I didn't interview Douglas Coupland, I interviewed myself. And I was unforgiving.

At the risk of making what might appear to be an unfair comparison (the life and health of a world-famous artist and author vs. that of a younger man climbing the creative class ladder), what follows is a story told to me by D, a friend who lives a very different life from the one Douglas Coupland describes. Coupland would like D, I suspect, and D is a Coupland fan. They are both go-getters. I have changed the names and places in this true story to protect my friend D, who still works for the agency, and the clients described below.

D is employed in a high-ranking position with an international advertising agency. He lives in a large Canadian city. He works constantly: nights, weekends and holidays. It's how he got to where he is today, and he's well compensated for his efforts. Almost forty, he has worked in marketing and advertising for over a decade. And, it's important to note, he loves his work.

One of D's clients is a multinational fast-food chain owned by a conglomerate, and he is responsible for a large chunk of their Canadian advertising. He comes up with advertisements and campaigns, catchy slogans, and directs the filmed ads as well as the online content. The client is demanding, as most clients in his business are, and also very much function on a Twenty-Four-Hour Workday schedule – a premise they expect their hired help to accept and remain in sync with.

A few months before I began writing this book, D had a brief but intense mental and physical collapse. The path to that collapse was unique and personal, of course, and D admits that he often pushes himself too hard, but what is not unique about his narrative is how the expectations of his employers, expectations they considered perfectly reasonable, contributed to his breakdown (for which he was never compensated, despite telling his immediate bosses the alarming details).

D began a typical day with a flight from his hometown to a smaller Canadian city about four hours away by air. His flight took off at 5 a.m., which meant being at the airport at 3:30 a.m. He had worked until nine or ten the night before. He arrived at the job site, a film studio, and worked on a new commercial for the fast-food chain.

The day dragged on, but that was typical. Film shoots always take twice as long as planned. D was used to that, and built the extra time into his agenda. The commercial was finally done and ready for editing, which would take place in D's home city. He flew back on a 6 p.m. flight, all the while answering text messages from his main employer, the advertising heads from the fast-food chain, and the people involved in the film shoot. He only turned his phone off when he had to, once the plane was in the air.

D arrived at home, said hello to his partner and ran back out the door. He had promised to attend a friend's concert and, being in a band himself, didn't want to disappoint his pals, despite the fact that he had only slept a few hours before his flight early that morning. On the subway to the concert, he answered more texts from all the people – about a dozen – connected with the film shoot and the larger commercial campaign. D arrived at the concert around 11 p.m. and got a drink. The bar was packed and noisy, and his friend's band is an old-school heavy metal band – loud is never loud enough.

D's phone continued to vibrate and light up. (When I asked him why he didn't turn it off, he looked at me like he was a surgeon in the middle of a delicate operation and I had just asked him to step away from the body. 'I never turn it off,' he said.) The concert blasted on. At around 1 a.m., D got an email from the restaurant chain's head of marketing, a message several hundred words long detailing everything the marketing head thought wrong with the first rushes he'd been sent of the commercial finished only hours before. Half-awake at this point, D thought the email had come from his primary employer, and he wrote back that it was past midnight and what did his boss expect him to do at that hour?

Then D realized the email had come from the chain's marketing head and not his boss. He spent half an hour sending texts, attempting to calm the angry adman. (A note here: the time difference between where the marketing chief lived and where D lives is only three hours, so it was at least 11 p.m. when the chief started text-hollering – one imagines the chief works all hours on principle as well.)

It was close to 2 a.m. when D stepped into the men's room to collect his thoughts and send out another message to the cranky client. He had had only two drinks, both light beers. D stood in a stall, dug his humming phone out of his pants pocket, and then, in his words, 'I woke up on the floor with the bouncer looking over my face and asking me my name.'

D passed out again. When he woke up once more, he was vaguely aware that the bouncer was still talking to him and that his pants were damp from the pissed-on floors. D lost consciousness a third time. The bouncer lifted him up, and D awoke, and then went under again. This pattern carried on for fifteen or twenty minutes, with the bouncer, who assumed D was blind drunk, trying to lift him up and get him to hold on to the stall walls. D could not lift himself or make his legs work.

The bouncer, and now a small crowd, began to talk about calling an ambulance. D came to long enough to tell the bouncer he was not drunk; he was having some sort of attack.

The bouncer, who, D says, 'was a giant, and a lamb,' asked D what he wanted to do. D opted to be gently shoved into a taxi and somehow, he is still not certain how, tell the driver his address. D phoned his partner, who met him at the bottom of the stairs to their apartment and pulled D inside. D's partner wanted to call an ambulance, but D only wanted to sleep. D's partner told me she thought he must have fallen and was worried he had a concussion. D woke up for a bit and calmed his partner, who helped him into bed. He slept all the next day.

'The entire time this went down,' D tells me, 'my phone kept going off. Even at 3 a.m. My partner shut it off sometime around four. When I woke up a day later, there were fifty-six messages, most from the client, some from my boss. At some point I guess I texted the client and said I was very tired, or that it was very late, something like that, but the client kept sending more ideas, more revisions, more questions about the commercial – and it was the middle of the night in the client's part of the world too.

'Nobody wrote anything about taking a break and waiting a few hours,' D continues, 'especially me – I was completely prepared to work at 1 a.m. and fix the situation if I could. It didn't seem unnatural or abusive, but perfectly normal, because that's my standard work pattern. And, the other irony, the project had an open-ended deadline – there was no urgency.

'Until I passed out, until my body and brain completely shut down, I didn't question why I thought it was reasonable to be answering work emails, massive emails, on my phone, in a bar, at a heavy metal concert, at 1 a.m. That's fucked.'

When D got back to his office, he told his boss the whole story, and apologized for missing a day's worth of texts and emails. His boss told D to take better care of himself, and instituted a new, less invasive policy regarding after-office-hours messaging: anything after 10 p.m. can wait.

'Ten o'clock at night,' D sighs. 'And my boss is a great guy, totally easy to work with. He's the Dream Boss type people want to work with – but even for him, expecting me to be awake enough to work, and do a good job, at 10 p.m., after working all day, is totally reasonable and totally ordinary. And I do it. It's like nobody learned anything from that incident. I was on the fucking floor and unconscious, but today I'm still answering messages way past 10 p.m. I don't know whose fault this is anymore.

'The other messed up part is that the entire time, from leaving the airport to going to the bar, I was tired, dead tired, but I kept going because the "rational" part of my brain kept telling me I could sleep later, or I didn't need sleep, or that I couldn't be a wuss and let sleep stop me from seeing my buddy's show.

'And when I came out of it,' continued D, who is thirty-nine, 'my first thought was "I am fucking getting old," not "Nobody can do this" or "This is not healthy." I still think that way; I passed out to the point where people thought maybe I was dying, but I still partly think it's my fault – for being older, for not being able to keep up, for needing sleep. Like an old man or a baby. I hate it. Sleep is still something I think of as … I don't know exactly … as like a waste, like an extravagance. Does that make any sense?'

D's phone goes off twice while we're talking, at 9:30 on a Friday night. Both messages are work-related.

Of course it is not the smart phones that keep us alert, it is our belief that we need to be alert all the time and the smart phones and other devices make that possible. If the candy is put in front of you, you will most likely grab and eat it. Anything that makes life easier for us is a welcome invention. But you pay a price. Because of cars, we are walking less. Because of smart phones, we sleep less. Both inventions make our lives more comfortable

and our work and communication faster, maybe even more effi-
cient. But we pay a price for that.

Temporarily I may neglect sleep for professional or private
occasions. But if I neglect it for too long, I tend to get thrown
out of balance. I start to feel nervous, my body may ache like I
have a fever … my whole emotional and physical resilience will
be affected.

I have learned about my boundaries and that it is better to
respect them in the long run.

— Dr. Med. Samia Little Elk, *Somnologin*, Berlin

D's story is alarming. What he describes is a work condition
and a set of work philosophies that support the systemic abuse
of the worker's health and also, perhaps more menacingly, are
so insidious that the worker learns to read the damaging work
ethic as not only natural and necessary, but as effective and
even enjoyable, a kind of endurance race with large rewards
for those who reach the finish line.

But what struck me most about D's story was that he
works in a creative industry that allows him no time to reflect,
to be still and think — an essential need for anyone who
employs their imagination. Reflection and observation, quiet
time, not only allow the mind to rest, but also create a fluid
mental space useful for observing a project as a whole, not
merely the sum of its parts, and to make connections between
the larger world and the project — connections easily overlooked during 'line by line' work.

D, a highly paid worker in a competitive creative field, has
no time to daydream, to gather inspiration from less immediate
sources, to step away from the project at hand. It would be
ironic, this depiction of a creative-class worker who has no
time to dream, no time for untasked creativity, were it not
so sad.

As Jonathan Crary remarks in *24/7*:

One of the forms of disempowerment within 24/7 environments is the incapacitation of daydream or of any mode of absent-minded introspection that would otherwise occur in intervals of slow or vacant time. Now one of the attractions of current systems and products is their operating speed: it has become intolerable for there to be waiting time while something loads or connects. When there are delays or breaks of empty time, they are rarely openings for the drift of consciousness in which one becomes unmoored from the constraints and demands of the immediate present. There is a profound incompatibility of anything resembling reverie with the priorities of efficiency, functionality, and speed.

The very systems that demand (and profit from) the spontaneous creativity of their workers are at the same time negating spontaneity and the generation of new ideas by erasing the 'openings,' as Crary puts it, wherein the mind wanders off the immediate task or situational problem to gain inspiration. In the fantasy world of the 24/7 economy, the production model is a perpetual motion machine that somehow runs without fuel. Eventually, the motor will grind to a shattering stop.

The Commodification of Sleep

On capitalism as disease and cure

Before I parade some of the more ridiculous 'insomnia cures' I've uncovered, I need to be honest about my own participation in the insomnia industry. I've tried everything, twice. The commodification of sleep horrifies me not because I look down on the consumers of these products as rubes, but because it is horrifying to consider that we are now entering an age wherein sleep can be and is sold. Quacks selling tonics have been around as long as the concept of curing – what we have today is the positioning of sleep as a commodifiable resource, a natural function supplied by our bodies that many of us must now buy back and then give back to our bodies. The head of the international conglomerate Nestlé Foods has declared that 'water is not a human right.' Nestlé sells bottled water. Is sleep the next basic human need to be repackaged as a product?

The consumerization of sleep is already on, and doing very well, but the products remain limited in their pitches to specialty markets (people with specific ailments, such as sleep apnea and lower back pain) or to the 'occasional' sufferer of sleeplessness (who is sold over-the-counter medications and bales of herbal teas). A casual look at the vendors who rent space at sleep and sleep-medicine conferences resembles a peek into a seventeenth-century curio cabinet of weird contraptions and weirder promises.

The annual SLEEP Conference, a U.S.-based event that describes itself as the 'premiere sleep medicine event of the year,' offers among its Reasons to Attend the promise that attendees will 'learn crucial business strategies.' Past exhibitors include Dream Water, which is exactly what it sounds like, an infused water to be taken before sleep, alleged to block 'the transmission of impulses from one cell to another in the central nervous system' via the inclusion of naturally sourced '5-HTP... [the] immediate nutrient precursor to the neurotransmitter, serotonin, which relays signals between brain cells ... and helps to reestablish healthy sleep patterns in people with sleep disturbances'; Pad A Cheek, which is nowhere near as sexy as it sounds, but is actually a line of padding products to better enhance one's sleep-apnea-mask experience (their slogan: 'Just because we have to wear a MASK all night doesn't mean we have to wear the MARKS all morning'); Re-Timer sleep glasses, from Australia, a 'light device' worn like a pair of goggles that 'produces 100 per cent UV-free green light,' which, when applied, will give the wearer 'the freedom to fall asleep and wake up when you choose'; and Sleepio, an online service that assesses your needs through a series of questionnaires and then applies cognitive behavioural therapy, taught via a cute cartoon virtual sleep expert called the Prof, to fix your sleep problems (the program also includes the Thought Checker application, to make sure you are teaching yourself how to sleep and better organize your sleeping schedule). And that's only a small handful of the 110-plus vendors and exhibitors listed.

Granted, the above are some of the more silly-appearing vendors. But given that the conference makes no distinction between vendors selling cranes to hold up your sleep-apnea-mask hose or 'intelligent beds,' and such major players as Lippincott, Williams & Wilkins, a venerable textbook and medical publishing conglomerate (founded in 1792), and the U.S. wing of Radiometer, a global medical-testing-device maker founded in 1935 in Copenhagen with a specialty in blood gas analysis (now available in over one hundred countries), it is impossible for the untrained consumer to discern between the magic-bean hawkers and the medical breakthroughs.

Nor, perhaps, are we meant to – although apparently anyone can register to attend the conference (no credentials are requested for pre-registration), the 436-page abstracts of papers presented include the titles 'Orexin-1 Receptor Blockade Dysregulates REM Sleep in Pharmacological or Genetic Models of Orexin-2 Receptor Inhibition,' 'The Effect of Napping on the Diurnal Secretory Pattern of Cortisol in Toddlers' and 'The Effects of Gabapentin Enacarbil on Individual Items of the International Restless Legs Scale' ...

I point out these obscure and daunting titles not (just) to make easy fun, but to show how remote sleep medicine is from its clients, the actual under-slept public, in contrast to, for instance, pain medicine or weight/body-size medicine. While anxiety over sleep patterns has never been higher, sleep medicine has not reached pop culture status. Sleep disorders do not have celebrity advocates, as fitness does, or celebrity activists, like the push for medical marijuana. Insomniacs do not have chat-show heroes, a Dr. Oz or a Deepak Chopra. We don't even have Debbie Travis or Mike Holmes fixer-uppers.

Until sleep disorders are commercialized to the point of being the subject of reality television and other vehicles of mass therapy, sleeplessness will remain the domain of the highly specialized and the highly suspect. What sleep medicine needs, on a cultural level, is mainstreaming. This is critical because insomnia has become a class issue. Granted, I say that about everything – but multiple statistical studies cross-indicate that people in disadvantaged socio-economic circum-stances are the most likely to experience insomnia symptoms.

Although it looks primarily at variances and conflicts in statistical models of insomnia studies, the article does note that 'socioeconomic inequalities' are 'prospectively associated with later insomnia' and, although the previous studies cited lacked enough long-term information, and insomnia itself varies in description and symptoms, there is a probability that 'people with consistently poor sleep may have experienced daytime fatigue, impairing work performance and making it difficult to obtain or retain higher status jobs.' The study also shows that even with all variant factors counted, women are more likely to suffer from insomnia than men. Since women still make less money than men, the gender difference is also a class difference.

At this point, I could insert a vigorous argument for government assistance, call for a full-on Royal Commission – an arm-long list of recommendations trotted out during a sombre press conference. I would heartily endorse such an endeavour, and it might even be of some value, other than entertainment, but I am too tired, literally, and so are the rest of us insomniacs. Government interventions are slow, overcalculated and often ignored. We can't wait. So I am going to go against every fibre of my socialist self and wonder what would happen if we let the free market fix the problem? I realize that contradicts my mockery of the wacky products being sold to the sleepless, but I am positing that, in the short term, a well-monitored intervention by the private sector might provide some relief.

The post-unionist, post-labour-laws free market that demands a twenty-four-hour worker will soon realize a twenty-four-hour worker is not a profitable worker, that an exhausted person cannot 'compete in the global market,' as the high prayer goes. But global capital is hardly going to self-impose a new generation of workers' rights on its own abundance. What global capital will do, quickly and cheaply (granted, at some other set of hapless workers' expense), is sell us sleep. It is not hard to imagine a future wherein sleep-enhancing outlets, cheap and plentiful, will be as commonplace (and socially acceptable to use) as fitness gyms or meditation centres, and provide access to easy-to-use and easy-to-understand therapies. A complete reversal of insomnia culture will take generations, and much regulation.

Or the free market might sell us back the same daily rest we once understood to be a birthright. Yes, this is a shitty solution, but here's how it might play out: a mass, downward spiral in worker productivity is directly linked to sleep deprivation. Then, corporations manufacture sleep aids that actually work – from better mattresses to stronger medications – and workers buy the devices at a premium. Inevitably, cheaper and cheaper copies of the most popular and effective sleep aids become available. Thus, the free market is perceived to have corrected the problem.

That every single step along the way described above is fraught with problems, I am well aware. Sleep, like other basic human needs, such as water and air, has already been well commoditized, and, like sustenance, those who can't pay don't get what they need. But if we have learned anything from the Great Crash of 2008, it is that neo-liberal, unfettered markets do not change, even when change could work in their favour. Why, then, would I put any faith in such a system? Because what late capitalism does understand, and excels at, is the quick fix, which is really the quick sell. Why should anyone suffering from chronic sleeplessness take the high road and wait for a massive environmental and sociological – not to mention legislative and regulatory – shift and refuse a quick fix to appease some unattainable or prohibitively expensive ideal of holistic wellness?

Put simply: after decades of not sleeping properly, I am not asking too many questions about who stitched my new mattress, or whether or not chemical residues from the pills I take will end up in the aquifers. I don't have that luxury. Leaving the problem of insomnia in the uncareful hands of the free market is not a sustainable solution, and it pains me to argue for such a strategy – but insomnia culture itself is inherently unsustainable, and increasingly feels more and more like an elastic band stretched to the snapping point. Sustainable solutions are a luxury for cultures in crisis. Sometimes you have to fight fire with fire.

The parallel with obesity issues is useful here. When the medical industry began to warn parents about the dangers of childhood obesity, the market instantly introduced reduced-sugar treats, better play equipment and for-rent child activity venues. The Canadian government, meanwhile, took a decade to introduce a simple tax credit for enlisting one's children in sports.

The Economist recently published a fascinating examination of how people perceive time use – or misperceive it:

> In the corporate world, a 'perennial time-scarcity problem' afflicts executives all over the globe, and the matter has only grown more acute in recent years ... [W]hen people are paid more to work, they tend to work longer hours, because working becomes a more profitable use of time. So the rising value of work time puts pressure on all time. Leisure time starts to seem more stressful ... the time people spend at their desks is often seen as a sign of productivity and loyalty ...

Intriguingly, in this article, 'leisure time,' time away from work, is analyzed, but sleep, and the possible economic damage of not setting aside time to sleep, indeed of living in a world where one must set aside time for a natural function, is not discussed at all. The piece deconstructs itself by constantly reminding the reader that while it may not be healthy to live with less 'leisure time,' it sure is profitable. As the article notes, 'This extra time in the office pays off.'

Only when productivity is measurably threatened by the unreality of the Twenty-Four-Hour Workday will the same mechanisms that bought into the illusion of the never-sleeping worker produce fast and affordable countermeasures. Because, of course, profits threatened by drained workers can be rebuilt selling sleep aids to those same workers. Yes, this is a cynical diagnosis, and yes, I am advocating for a quick fix, a dollar-store cure, and yes, I recognize that as free-market-generated social cures play out over a generation they will ultimately eat themselves, the build-and-destroy cycle being a generative of late-capitalist profits ... But I can't go on like this, night after night, and neither can you. I'll fix the planet when I'm better.

> I was given generic Xanax to help me sleep and deal with anxi-ety, although it's addictive so I wasn't prescribed very much. It's great for short-term problems, and when taken with pot feels pretty great. I was also put on an SSRI that is supposed to alleviate OCD; it had terrible side effects and I hated it, so I went back to doing pot every day and I'm looking into Transcendental Meditation as a way to control impulses and sleep better. Because I am poor and have no insurance, I can't afford the cognitive behavioural therapy that can treat my problems, unless I go on a waiting list that can take up to two years before I see a professional. So in the meantime, pot is cheaper than anything else and that is how I get to sleep every night. In other words, I am batshit cray-cray, but I've embraced it.
>
> – L, Toronto

A side note: I have tried practically every over-the-counter pill, pillow and gentle plinking noise machine you can name. None of them work. I suspect they are still available for sale because most, if not all, of their buyers are first-and-last-time customers. It's the promises they make that are so alluring, not the payoff. My own pile of discarded non-cures may well constitute a solid case against the free-market solution, but I will argue that because sleep disorders lack the same presence in pop-culture dialogues around health and wellness as weight and fitness, better and reliable cures have not been invented due to the lack of a properly understood and identified market.

And I will never stop trying the latest wonder drugs or barley-shell pillows, because at least when I am buying something I think will help, I temporarily, semi-delusionally, feel that I have agency over my sleep disorder, that I can be proactive, a wallet warrior. Fleeting peace of mind is still peace of mind.

One of the more insidious aspects of insomnia culture is the escalation factor built into the use of prescribed medication and the abuse of self-medication. After a relatively short while, in terms of a life span, the prescribed medications cease to work as well, if at all. I suspect once one goes about rewiring one's brain chemistry artificially, there is a Newtonian reaction in the brain that results in a further but different rewiring.

And so, one has to take a new, stronger medication or more of the initial, but now less functional, medication. Self-medicators face parallel problems, with upped dosages of their favourite legal or illegal cures. We use the language of 'addiction' to describe these patterns, but is it fair to describe the fallout from a systemic failure in sleep health as an addiction, a term loaded with moral implications and a subset of judgments and assessments relating to the user's 'will power' and supposed lack of inner strength – and that reading of the insomniac's subsequent addictions does nothing more than mirror and buttress her already nagging innate sense that she cannot sleep because she lacks discipline, a well-balanced life, healthy habits, etc.

The unsuitability of confronting a broad public health problem with addicting chemicals by sponsoring and industrializing the ensuing addictions (or by ignoring the larger, pandemic-like problem in the hopes that sufferers will simply self-medicate themselves into a stupor for long enough each day to remain functional) is gallingly thoughtless and arguably abusive. Every system to date that claims to aid insomniacs eventually turns on the client-patients, making them unwell in new ways, ways that cannot be just coincidentally highly compatible with insomnia itself. The failure of contemporary culture and its health industries to address chronic sleep issues surpasses wilful ignorance, which, arguably, could be read as somewhat innocent, and slides into absentee malevolence, or at least negligence, when these failures foster further, easily lethal health problems.

On doctors, doctors and more doctors

I start my nightly obsession with not sleeping early, often at 10 p.m. and sometimes as early as the morning before. I know insomnia. It is my constant companion. Very often after a few hours my mind is alert enough that when I wake up it races, thinks about all the things I did not do in the day, all the people I did not contact. I often read between 3 and 5 a.m. – fiction – which soothes my mind and my heart but does a disservice to the careful reading of the fiction. I have my sleep cocktails ranging from valerian to anti-anxiety medication to plain old Aspirin. Night is for demons and catastrophizing.

– K, Chicago

I never stop trying, and though I am often grouchy and approach medical consultations with a chip the size of a refrigerator on my shoulder, a habit I find not only reprehensible but also just plain churlish, I still go, I still ask questions, I still try to fix my sleep health. Insomniacs are the bitchiest optimists in the world.

My latest sleep clinic and sleep doctor, first visited in November 2014, are located in Toronto's north end, a ninety-minute bus ride from downtown. Everyone on the bus is yawning. But that's the public transit norm in Toronto – I can't blame insomnia for everything.

Conversely, the clinic is the happiest medical facility I have ever visited. Everybody knows everybody else and the gossiping and symptom-sharing is relentless. 'Can you believe he's still alive? And doing his own groceries!' 'He's a miracle on legs, I'm telling you.' 'Who are you seeing today? Doctor ____ is very nice! I had him last week.' Etc.

As you can likely guess, everyone in the waiting room is well over sixty-five, and I can tell they are checking me out, wondering what could possibly be wrong with somebody, anybody, under the age of fifty. I'm in my prime; I should not be bothering doctors.

The doctors, however, are all under forty and incredibly genial. They hug their patients and shake their hands. They ask after the patients' pets and grandchildren. And, typical of Toronto, the room is a mix of people from many heritages: older Jews who have lived in the Bathurst-and-Steeles neighbourhood for a lot longer than the clinic has been in existence; Chinese twentysomethings escorting their grandmothers; cute, beefy Polish guys waiting to drive their dads home; a Portuguese receptionist with an enormous top knot and tight leggings that delight the older gents, who indiscreetly peek over her high desk; and one Indo-Canadian man close to my age who puts his asthma puffer to his lips like a cigar.

I'm not much of a booster, civic or otherwise, but you really don't see this sort of assembly anywhere else on earth. I'm happy to be here, happy to watch the human parade.

My doctor is under thirty-five, Asian-Canadian and sweet-tempered. He instantly recognizes that I am one frustrated medical client, and drops the basic questions, the ones I first answered years ago (is your bedroom dark at night, is your bedroom quiet at night, do you read in bed, is your bedroom stuffy, do you drink coffee four hours before bedtime, do you have a regular bedtime …).

He also realizes I am well past covering the sleep-hygiene basics and moves directly to the question of insomnia and restless leg syndrome. On the rare nights when I am not kicking myself awake over and over, I tell him, complete with re-enactments of the more furious styles of kicking that my legs have perfected, I simply don't fall asleep.

We talk about breathing. There is nothing wrong with my breathing. He takes my blood pressure, which runs a little high and has for years. We talk more about my breathing. He looks me over and I understand where he is going with his questions. I'm overweight. Obesity and sleep apnea have a causal relationship. But I don't have sleep apnea. Nevertheless, my nice doctor starts telling me about an exciting new diet developed by one of his clients (the diet is little more than an updated version of the now-unfashionable Atkins Diet, which I point out to him, but he dodges the question).

A few more minutes wasted on diet chat (I took a ninety-minute bus ride for three minutes of sleep consultation and ten minutes of diet chat?), and I ask him bluntly if there is any science linking body size and RLS. No, there is not, he says. Fine, thanks, I say, let's stop talking about diets. I've been fat since I was ten, longer than he's been alive; he has nothing to tell me about diets. When you are fat, doctors will read any and every thing wrong with your health through the gummy lenses of your body size.

At this point, the nice doctor begins to realize he is dealing with a chronic patient, one who's been through the sleep-medicine mill. He looks over the chart provided by my regular doctor.

'You're taking clonazepam for RLS?'

For about twenty years now, I tell him.

'Then, then – you're dependent on it!'

So what? Better dependent than dead.

He hmms and harumphs a bit, and suddenly, out of nowhere, mentions a drug I have never heard of, drops the name of this drug as casually as one might mention Aspirin.

Mirapex, 0.25 milligrams, taken thirty minutes before bed, to block the neurological triggers of RLS.

A miracle drug! I'm about to cry.

'It's been around for about a decade,' he continues.

What? What? A decade? I have never, ever heard of Mirapex.

'It's the most common drug for RLS,' he says, again with that 'Have an Aspirin' tone.

Common? I'm astounded. In all my trolling of RLS forums and nagging every doctor who's had the misfortune to meet me, including my dentist and her hygienist, Mirapex has not come up.

'You take it once a day'.

So, it's the cure … the cure…

'No, there is no cure. Mirapex is just for relief.'

Side effects?

None.

Counter-indications with my current prescriptions?

None.

How long will I need to take it?

'Oh, it's a chronic usage drug – for life, in other words.'

'In other words, I'll be dependent on it,' I retort.

He shrugs.

As for a sleep test, the full overnight visit with electrodes, he tells me there is no need. Sleep tests only catch respiratory problems.

'We videotape them,' he says, 'so we'd see that you have RLS, but you already know you have RLS, so why bother?'

I am relieved by this news. But I am also wondering why, again, I am being given contrary information, being told that sleep tests only monitor sleep apnea?

Did doctors in the past simply look at my body size and assume I have breathing difficulties? I used to make the joke when I suffered from mild seasonal allergies that I now had all the ingredients to make me the character Piggy from *Lord of the Flies* – chubby body, glasses and 'asthmar.'

Were all my previous doctors in on the gag? Furthermore, and more important, I'm frightened of this new drug. I don't believe anything powerful enough to rearrange my brain chemistry (and I know from powerful brain-changing pills) does not have side effects, counter-indications, at least trigger a bad headache. I agree to try the drug, but for a week only, and not until my regular doctor returns from his vacation, in case something goes wrong.

I also promise myself I will not look up the drug online, not frighten myself, will give Mirapex an honest try. As for the dependency issue, well, what's one more drug?

'How much does it cost?' I ask. (I always ask doctors how much medications cost, having no insurance plan that covers medications – and they always respond the same way: 'No idea' – and why would they know, they've got cupboards full of freebies).

My young sleep doctor looks at me like I've asked him for the exact price, with taxes, of a flight from Toronto to Johannesburg. He has no idea.

Mirapex (SDZ-Pramipexole DI-HCL Monohy 0.25mg, to be precise) is not a wonder drug. It is barely a drug at all, according to my body. I am both disappointed and not surprised. I've been down Promise Road before, and up and down Try Again Path.

The side effects – remember, I was told there would be none – include constipation and its vibrant opposite, constant thirst and a caked, dry mouth, headaches, vivid nightmares, compulsive eating (and purging, which I am already prone to during times of high stress) and, worst of all, only very minimal relief from RLS. I'm glad I didn't look Mirapex up on the internet – some patients fall asleep in the middle of sentences and have hallucinations! I got off easy.

The first night I took Mirapex, I felt nothing. I twitched and kicked like the old pro I am. The second night, my legs were happy to rub together repeatedly but not kick. The third night, I actually passed out, felt doped and heavy-headed. The fourth night, my legs were back in action.

I had a week's worth of test pills (at about $2.20 a pill), and by the end of the week the RLS had rerouted the new chemicals in my brain and wholly defeated their minor intrusion. I am not taking Mirapex again.

I can hear the arguments for taking Mirapex again: such as *I need a stronger dose, or I need to try it for a longer period of time, or I need to experiment with what time of day I take the dose*, etc. But I know my own body, and I know that if I got to a dosage of Mirapex that actually worked reliably, I would need it forever (which I have no moral problem with: addictions are manageable), and I would need to take more powerful doses over time.

Rather, I will wait for a cure. I am tired of band-aids and plasters. And if the cure never comes, at least I can spend the extra $60 to $100 a month on things that amuse me.

There is another, more ominous subtext to my rejection of Mirapex: Parkinson's disease. Mirapex's use as a treatment for RLS is secondary to its primary use, as a drug therapy for people suffering from tremors and Parkinson's-inflicted shakiness. I suspect any benefits for RLS were discovered by accident.

Parkinson's disease comes up constantly when one discusses RLS with doctors or reads about RLS. I'm haunted by Parkinson's. Am I living in a pre-Parkinson's state? Will drugs that attach themselves to the neurochemicals that inflict Parkinson's disease further the progress of the disease, or is that unscientific, homeopathic thinking, a sympathetic magic delusion?

I'm frightened that I am going to develop Parkinson's, mostly because my medical advisors keep mentioning it, ever so casually, as if they are about to suggest I be tested for the disease. I'm so terrified of Parkinson's that I've convinced myself that not taking a Parkinson's-indicated medicine will somehow ward off Parkinson's, keep me clear of the curse. And if RLS is a precursor to Parkinson's, I will simply end my life.

I'm not being dramatic, just factual. I do not want to live with Parkinson's, no thank you. I cannot imagine a life of any value being lived with that disease. I don't care if that is offensive to Parkinson's survivors, battlers or whatever they call themselves (or what I'd call myself). Life has value only in its quality. Being alive is simply not enough.

While I was writing this book, my dear mother, Dorothy, died. She was in her late eighties and had had cancer for over a year. She tried chemotherapy and it nearly killed her. My brother and I sat with her in her doctor's office on the day she decided, rather bluntly, to stop taking chemotherapy.

She looked up at the doctor, who was pushing for 'another round' of poison (nine weeks' worth, no less) and, bright as a candle, said, 'No.' Just 'No.'

I understood her completely. Better to live out the time she had left in relative comfort than to fight a miserable fight against the inevitable, to carry on for the sake only of carrying on, with all the vomit and the bed-shitting and the wrenching, spinning horror of chemotherapy. I respect my mother's decision; I admire her for her reasonable approach to life. Life is to be lived, not endured. Life is so very much more than mere breathing and digesting, infinitely more than the cycling and recycling of fluids and oxygen. And it is up to the person living that life to decide when to stop.

If I develop Parkinson's disease, if all these years of sleeplessness have been a preamble to that particular hell, then I too will say 'No,' gladly.

A side note. After trying and writing about Mirapex, I stumbled a few weeks later, in January 2015, on what appeared to be a 'placed' article (i.e., one dictated or driven by a public relations agency) on the website RLS.org. The article detailed how Mundipharma, a multinational, multi-tiered pharmaceutical concern that, according to its own website, provides 'fully integrated, strategic support and services to individual companies within the Mundipharma network' and 'help[s] our partners gain approval from regulators and build markets for their products,' had just announced that it had been given clearance by the European Commission to release its drug Targin 'as a second line symptomatic treatment for patients with severe to very severe idiopathic restless legs syndrome (RLS), after failure of dopaminergic therapy.' Targin is the trade name Mundipharma uses for its brand of oxycodone, a highly addictive painkiller. And it is the first opioid to be given a licence in the European Union for treatment of RLS.

In North America, where oxycodone (or 'hillbilly heroin,' as it is popularly derided) addiction is highest, and the subject of much hand-wringing by legal, drug regulation and medical institutions alike, reading that oxycodone – even a prolonged-release version of the drug, as Targin is – has been proposed to treat a chronic condition like RLS is terrifying. Is this the best the medical industry can do for RLS sufferers: stun us with opioids? And don't forget the side effects, which include '[a]n adverse event profile for oxycodone/naloxone over the entire study period that was consistent with the safety profile of opioids.' Translation: it's addictive, very addictive – combined with 'gastrointestinal disorders, headache, somnolence, fatigue, pruritus [itching], and hyperhidrosis [excessive sweating].'

A drug to treat a sleep disorder that leaves you sleepy and fatigued is either a moronic stab in the dark, a cynical cash grab or a brilliant counterintuitive gesture. There is desperation to this drug therapy that sadly mimics the tone of a typical insomniac's life, and the larger insomnia culture. As I proposed earlier, I am ready to take obviously unsustainable measures to cure my sleeplessness because the reality of living in an insomnia culture, as an insomniac, is unsustainable, so why not create compatible, if short-term, therapies? Nevertheless, the grim prescription of a high-grade opiate feels a bit like being told to visit an opium den.

To date, the drug is not approved for insomnia in Canada.

Cinq à Sept with Dr. Dang-Vu
On experts and alarm bells

Mostly my insomnia revolves around repetitive OCD thoughts. It's easier to distract myself from these thoughts during the day (although they do interfere with my day-to-day activities). It gets much worse at night, while lying in the dark with nothing to do. Pot has really helped in this department; although it doesn't always work, for the most part regular use has helped me get to sleep. Here's a sampling of the things that keep me awake: lock-checking is big: did I lock my bike, the building door, the apartment door, the shop door? I will get out of bed, put clothes on and check all of these. So-called 'Doom Thoughts': OCD-related brain junk like imagining horrible things happening to family members, pets, friends, etc. Accidents, illnesses, etc. General worry/anxiety: finances, exams, what am I doing with my life, etc. Recapping horrible things I have seen/heard about: sometimes my brain will just race through horrible things that I've seen or have happened to me. Accidents I've witnessed, animals being abused … The list is endless.

– L, Toronto

Judging from the raft of books and media coverage on sleeplessness currently available (one prominent doctor described insomnia as 'the new tobacco'), I am obviously not alone in my assertion that insomnia is no longer just a disorder, it's a way of life, sometimes even a chosen way of life. But what do the experts outside of pop medicine have to say? I needed to have an actual conversation with an actual expert, one who was not in any way involved in my own treatment or possible treatments – somebody who had nothing to gain or sell.

Dr. Thien Thanh Dang-Vu is a Montreal sleep specialist who graciously agreed to take an hour (and, as you'll learn, this man's spare hours are precious and far between) to answer my questions about insomnia and his particular field of sleep research.

A charming and handsome young intellectual, Dr. Dang-Vu works in a mid-century building that shares none of the same modifiers. I almost felt sorry for him, having to stare down that ugly space every day – until he casually (and without a hint of doctorish arrogance) ticked off his impressive CV.

'Tell me about you and your work,' I start, innocently enough.

'I am thirty-four years old. I have an MD (Neurology) from Université de Liège, Belgium, and a PhD in neuroscience. I did post-doctoral work in Boston Massachusetts General Hospital, and then the Université de Montréal (Sleep Centre). I'm an assistant professor at Concordia University (Exercise Science and Psychology) and a neurologist/clinical professor at Institute Universitaire de Gériatrie de Montréal/University of Montreal (Neurosciences). My practice is primarily research-based, but I see two or three patients per week, by referral.'

'Ummm. Wow.' I've been in his office less than five minutes and I feel like I have done nothing with my life. 'That's a lot of degrees for a thirty-four-year-old,' I blurt out.

Dr. Dang-Vu shrugs and smiles. He knows he's an over-achiever, perhaps even likes being one. I collect myself and forge ahead.

Dr. Dang-Vu goes on to describe the particular, and hyper-specific neurological disorders he studies, all of which lead to sleep disruption and sound perfectly terrifying. He describes his test subjects and how he conducts the tests, and I realize he is describing a basic sleep test. At this point, I'm feeling overwhelmed, but something in the back of my head jumps to the front. I have been told, repeatedly, that sleep tests only monitor sleep apnea, a respiratory disorder. What's all this neurological jazz?

'Oh, no,' Dr. Dang-Vu says, 'there are many neurological sleep problems that traditional sleep tests can catch. Research is looking at the brain causes of multiple sleep disorders and how they evolve to Parkinson's and other neurodegenerative disorders. So the tests are very important. But all of these disorders I'm listing, the common ones and the more rare ones, are testable. Traditional sleep tests can reveal many more conditions than the common sleep apnea. Insomnia research is at its heart the study and biological classification of insomnia – very heterogeneous condition – and of predictors of responses to treatments, in order to guide choice of therapeutic intervention. It's not all about sleep apnea.'

Now I'm starting to get angry. And there's the apparition of Parkinson's again, floating over Dr. Dang-Vu's desk. 'Why,' I ask, 'have I been told, many times, that sleep tests only catch sleep apnea?'

Here, Dr. Dang-Vu decides to opt for a diplomatic response. 'There are many other disorders of sleep than sleep apnea. For instance, insomnia is more common than apnea; about 15 per cent of the population has chronic insomnia disorder. REM Sleep Behaviour Disorder and narcolepsy require a sleep test in lab for the diagnosis … but apnea benefited from more attention possibly because the medical industry has moved its focus and technology to treating apnea due to the commercial developments … Many forms of insomnia disorder can, however, be effectively treated, without the need of technology or drugs.'

I won't put words into Dr. Dang-Vu's mouth, but from my own research it is apparent to me that the sleep apnea treatment business is enormously profitable (the sleep masks, the accessories for the sleep masks, the nose clips, the special pillows and mechanized mattresses, you name it), and so of course clinics and clinicians are chasing the money. I don't have to be diplomatic; I'm not a doctor.

I realize this line of questioning is making Dr. Dang-Vu uncomfortable, so I move on. 'Why is insomnia so culturally prevalent?'

'There are two elements,' Dr. Dang-Vu begins. 'One is the increased awareness of the disorder – although it is important to note that there are distinct cultural differences at play: some cultures simply ignore insomnia and dismiss it; for instance, in Asia a decade ago, nobody in the medical field studied insomnia, and that is in many ways related to the lack of attention and culture of shame attached to psychiatry as well – especially in the West, where there is much more awareness now of insomnia. The second aspect is that there are now increased factors that promote sleep disorders – look at our culture of consumption, from how much we eat to how much we distract ourselves, and see how this has led to an increased prevalence of insomnia.'

Our culture of consumption, of course, is dependent on our fixation with productivity. Without non-stop productivity, there are not enough products to consume. It's a tidy circle. And a deadly one: we work more and sleep less so that we can acquire more, and many of the products we most treasure are designed to stimulate, or at least distract us, and that keeps us even more awake and alert – a state that is valued economically and can increasingly only be deflected (but rarely halted) with another type of over-consumption: namely, medication.

Dr. Dang-Vu reaffirms, 'We all work late, we all work faster and faster. Myself, I do this too. I am also guilty of this! All of this busyness keeps the brain awake and preoccupied, which obviously does not facilitate sleep. For instance: many people go to bed in a state of hyper-arousal, because of work or other distractions, and then in pre-sleep they cannot decrease their worries or intrusive thoughts. But people ignore this problem and will not or cannot change their daily habits.'

To maintain and build upon his already high status as a researcher and doctor, Dr. Dang-Vu must practice exactly the kind of poor sleep hygiene, and suffer its symptoms, that he has built a career on. If people employed in the sleep industry

– indeed, its upper echelons – find themselves frequently attempting sleep in a state of 'hyper-arousal,' what hope is there for the underemployed and people who work in less privileged positions? As Dr. Dang-Vu notes, the problem is systemic – people 'cannot' change their habits, because they lack the power to do so in their workplace, the power to demand more time for sleep – and psychological – workers 'will not' change their habits. The 'will' is the more insidious of the two. Our minds are being retrained to see sleep as a waste of time, but whose time? Not our own.

So, in medicine we prescribe pills to help calm the mind, but pills don't help in the long term. Pills induce dependency and the efficiency of the medications decrease with time, so you have to take more. But if we all live in this sped-up society, why would we not seek immediate relief, like the kind pills appear to offer?

'There are also sociological and class factors at play,' Dr. Dang-Vu explains. 'People in many work positions can't step away from their work. They do not have that power in their workplace. To employers, the non-stop worker appears in the short term to be profitable, and it appears profitable to force more difficult "efficiencies" on workers, but in the long term productivity decreases because workers are less alert and are suffering from mood disruptions, anxieties, poor concentration – this is very hazardous to people's physical health as well, and causes accidents. And, further on, many workers develop health problems in association with their poor sleeping lives, and those problems become a source of economic stress to employers and to public health. So, what is "efficiency"?'

Dr. Dang-Vu sits back in his chair and exhales. 'In my own life, I have lived this way too. I was a medical resident and had to do overnights, work for twenty-four to thirty-six hours non-stop, all the time trying to stay awake. Everybody knew it was not good for productivity, but they treated it, and still treat it, like an "initiation process."'

'Why,' I ask, 'has the medical industry not changed this outdated practice, especially since the hazards are so obvious?'

'Ha! That is a very good question.' I finally got a laugh out of the good doctor. 'I think partly,' he continues, 'because people have trouble altering what is perceived as a tradition. There is a culture of "sleep is wasteful," even among doctors, who know better!'

If even doctors are messing with their sleep health, that raises an obvious follow-up question: what happens to our bodies when we continue to live this way?

'Up to a certain point, our bodies adapt, which is why it is hard to recognize symptoms at first. We can convince ourselves that we are strong, that we need less sleep. But if you repeat this not-sleeping over and over, your body will be affected, of course, and your body changes in ways that you cannot perceive at first. For instance, one single night of not sleeping well can change your glucose metabolism, and if this happens again and again, it can become a factor in pre-diabetes. But nobody knows that – one night of bad sleep alters your glucose metabolism! That is just one night. Eventually the alterations in your body catch up with you. Consistent not-sleeping also can lead to hypertension. Those are just two of many problems that can develop from poor sleep. Living without enough sleep can't be sustained. It is the opposite of "productivity" in the long term.'

Diabetes and Parkinson's disease, in one conversation. Lucky, already-triggered me. I have to stop internalizing every bit of information …

Dr. Dang-Vu isn't sure where our insomnia-plagued culture is headed, but he believes it's possible to be productive and have good sleep hygiene too. 'People need to know that their brains are working while they sleep, and that those brain functions during sleep make you even smarter. Perhaps people also need to learn how to be more structured and organized. I know this is not a popular idea, but with sufficient organization and a bit of applied habit, you can minimize sleep problems – and I say that while admitting that I myself am the first person to be bad at what I am advising others to do.

'We always want to take on more. Right now, I am doing ten projects with students. To work this way, overwork, it's how I was educated and how I was taught to manage my career. Also, in research projects, you try to maximize your results by doing more, because not all projects work out. Some days I feel like I have four or even six jobs at the same time. I'm tired, but I work late too. And I know the consequences, but I do it anyway! I do things I would not recommend to my patients. I don't have insomnia, I can fall asleep, but I never have enough sleep.'

'If even you, a neurologist with expertise in sleep, are living, by your own design, without adequate sleep, doesn't that mean that insomnia is now normalized in our culture?' I ask, hoping for a negative response but knowing better.

'Well, we have to ask what is the norm first,' Dr. Dang-Vu replies, 'and I think that although insomnia might be normalized, so is having a nap. Napping is socially acceptable, not looked at as laziness. We are adapting our ideas of 'normal' regarding sleep. But it is hard to talk about insomnia in a thematic way, because there are so many types: is not falling asleep the new normal, or not staying asleep the new normal, or waking up too early the new normal? However, when any of these complaints are associated with their consequences, it is perhaps more exact to say society has normalized the symptoms of insomnia. And that is scary.

'The more immediate problem is the option most people take to fix their sleep hygiene – pills. Pills are the number one treatment, because there are very few available or affordable other options. Pills are not the best, but an entire life change is very hard to do for individuals and very slow and costly for the system to assist. How we perceive sleep needs to change. Cognitive behaviour therapy works very well with sleep disorders, but it requires active commitment and active assistance, and also we have very few well-trained specialists in cognitive behavior therapy for insomnia (CBTI). Furthermore, the cost of CBTI is not currently reimbursed by the provinces, because it is considered "psychology," not "real" health care. So, class issues appear again. Who can afford treatment?

'There is a lack of vision in our system,' Dr. Dang-Vu continues. 'We don't want to integrate different practices, even when they are proven to work, and we don't want to pay up front for something, even when not treating the disorder costs more money in the long run. So people take pills.'

'We know now that insomnia creates psychological problems too – you can have difficulty regulating or controlling your emotions. Insomniacs are very prone to "catastrophic thinking –"' oh, testify, doctor, testify! "– and then they have more trouble sleeping. Again, this is a cognitive problem. CBTI is very good at fixing this, and we have discovered that CBTI fixes other syndromes that are related to insomnia, such as depression. What you might call "pure insomnia" is very rare: there are usually other syndromes in play as well. Often people who seek out CBTI because they can't sleep realize that other problems, such as depression and anxiety, are also helped – problems they sometimes did not even realize they had until they started to work on their sleep.'

Being a chronic deconstructor, I have to ask: isn't it ironic that a possible solution to being chronically under-slept because of our warped 'productivity culture' is another system that requires, like CBTI, a labour-intensive practice from the patient?

'Yes, the irony is there,' Dr. Dang-Vu says with a chuckle, 'but these intensive and long-term solutions are a different kind of "work" – you are working toward relaxation and learning, teaching yourself to adopt behaviours that will reset your sleep ideas, your existing conditioning toward sleep, learning to start seeing the bed as a productive space too, and sleep as productive, not simply "crashing," which sounds like a failure. But CBTI-style therapies take a lot of patience, and people have to make an effort.'

Dr. Dang-Vu's free hour is coming to a close, so I end with a Big Picture question.

'If, as I believe, we are moving toward living full-time in an "insomnia culture," what will our world look like fifteen or twenty years from now?'

'If we don't change, we are in danger of counterbalancing the many advances we have made in health care,' Dr. Dang-Vu says flatly. 'We will become more vulnerable: to chronic disorders, to diseases, to disruptions in our health. One of the issues people don't understand, or are maybe just starting to understand, is that there are cost increases (of all kinds) to our becoming more vulnerable. Productivity has costs. Try to envision the already bad inequalities in our society increased enormously, and in more facets, than ever before. That could be what the world will look like. Everything that is a societal problem now will be a bigger problem.'

Oh, fuck. Well, what is to be done?

'We need to change our expectations of sleep,' says Dr. Dang-Vu, "and have a clearer perception of what sleep is and does. You can tell people over and over that sleep is important, but that sometimes makes them more anxious and then they can't sleep! I see this all the time with chronic insomniacs – they have an idea or ideas about how sleep is supposed to be, the idea that there are common practices of sleep that they are not partaking in – for instance, that everyone needs eight hours a night. This is not true. Everyone has different sleep needs, it varies widely from person to person, but insomniacs now have moved from making themselves anxious over not sleeping to making themselves anxious over "sleeping correctly." I hear this every day from patients: *I must have eight hours and I must go to bed every night at 10 p.m.*, or whatever the "rules" are. So the anxieties are growing layers.

'Genetics play a part in our sleep needs, our internal clocks play a part, our environments and cultures play a part and our personalities play a part. There is a simple math, though, that can be used as a general but not strict rule: if you have a lot of activities in your day, you have a higher sleep need; if you have a more passive day, then you have lower sleep needs. But that is a really simple starting point.

'You have to be attentive to the whole picture of your life when you consider your sleep practices. I'm describing a holistic approach while I am aware we are not living in a world that has much patience for holistic living of any kind!'

We say our goodbyes and I decide to walk to my temporary apartment in Montreal. The first snow has come and disappeared, and it is freezing cold outside; cold and dark, wet dark. Saint Joseph's Oratory towers over the neighbourhood like a massive spaceship, a floating, bubble-domed wonder of lights and reflected marble. The streets are almost bare, but the apartment blocks are busy hives.

Everyone appears to be at home, cooking or watching television or reading emails, savouring the warm indoors and their comforting distractions. It is a perfect night to go to bed early. But few will. I look back at Dr. Dang-Vu's office building. All of the office lights are on. Everybody is still working, still alert … as I too will be for hours to come.

The War on Sleep
On the confessions of a sleep doctor

I n my immediate family, there are four people in their twenties. The language they use to describe their sleep habits (another loaded phraseology) is telling. Nights when they must retire in order to be alert the next day are called 'school nights,' i.e., nights burdened by obligations and expectations forced upon them by inescapable and duty-binding systems. When they do stay up all night they describe how they 'power through' the following day, borrowing language from sports, as if being exhausted is the equivalent of winning a trophy. When sleeplessness finally catches up with them and their bodies shut down, they talk of 'crashing,' language borrowed from another set of more active, menace-laden metaphors.

The language they use to talk about sleep reflects their own distorted relationship with sleep – sleep is a chore, and yet sleep is also a treat, sleep is something to be conquered, a nagging requirement of the body that our starve-to-thrive culture tells them to defeat in order to succeed (the parallels with food intake and body-size readings are inescapable), yet at the same time sleep is obligatory, a tax to be paid, again, to ensure success. And the dilemma over sleep is made more melodramatic by being shared while lived, via instant communications. A disorder turned into an impulse, insomnia has yet to find its own original language.

In April 2014 (on April Fool's Day, tellingly), the government of France introduced a law that prevents employers from sending emails or other digitally generated messages to employees before 9 a.m. and after 6 p.m. The news of this new law spread fast, and became a lead story in business newspapers the next day. The law was hailed as a bold counterstrike against the debilitating effects of the Twenty-Four-Hour Workday, and was equally derided in pro-business circles as an impediment to international trade and/or as an example of unionism gone mad.

The thing is, the law never existed. Or, to be more precise, never existed in the form in which it was reported to exist (more on that later). But the story spread so widely and so fast that France's Minister for Digital Economy, Axelle Lemaire, was forced to issue a correction (via digital messaging – a tweet, naturally).

The actual legislative event was an agreement struck exclusively between employers and workers in the high tech and tech consulting fields – typically people who are in communication with co-workers around the world and are thus forced to work during the traditional off-hours of the nine-to-five schedule. The agreement protected barely a quarter of a million people, all of them soi-disant 'autonomous workers' (an adorably French, adorably hopeful term for us freelancers, the least protected yet most educated sloggers in the labour sector).

The complexities of the message-permission agreement are not worth repeating, especially since the rules around when employers are permitted to contact workers have nothing to do with the hour of the day, but rather how many hours a worker has already clocked on any given day. There never was a 6 p.m. cut-off or a 9 a.m. start time.

The 'no emails after 6 p.m.' story, however poorly understood and/or misreported, intrigued Western workers not because it was revealed to be an unintentional hoax, but because everyone who read and repeated the initial misinformation very much wanted the story to be true. We could almost envision it – a world where the evenings were ours again.

The venerable *Economist*, who initially reported the false story and then later corrected the report (two weeks later, on April 14, 2014), had a predictable London gentlemen's club response to the affair, sniping, 'The real trouble for France is that the story even appeared plausible in the first place.' Oh, how pithy! Unless you are a beleaguered 'autonomous worker' who sleeps with your phone by your bed.

Everyone I know sleeps with their phone by their bed, no matter their employment relationship, partly out of a fear of missing something, of being not available for real, life-or-death emergencies, but mostly because they are afraid of being perceived as poor workers, not ambitious enough for the new global economy.

Subsequently, everyone I know answers emails from work at 9 p.m., 11 p.m. ... 1 a.m. The boss is awake, the rationale goes, why aren't you? Aren't you a team player? What today's worker needs is not a complicated, and absolutely impossible-to-enforce, system of labour agreements and labour-code bylaws, but an overhaul of how our culture perceives and values sleep. Insomnia culture's productivity fantasias rely on citizens not demanding a right to rest as readily as they demand the basic (and interrelated) rights to food, shelter and personal security.

When sleep becomes a fundamental human right, as it must, insomnia culture will be read for what it so manifestly is: a naturalized systemic abuse supported by profit-chasing and myriad, deep social dysfunctions. Attempts to protect citizens from this abuse will no longer be dismissed with nanny-state jokes.

But getting to this point where we recognize that sleep is vital to the security of the person will take a monumental shift in perception. We no longer callously joke about starvation, homelessness, pollution or physical violence – so why is an attempt, even such a flawed and insufficient attempt as the one negotiated in France, to protect citizens from chronic sleep deprivation (a problem with an overabundance of medical information detailing its detriments) instantly met with waves of ridicule and perceived as further proof of the laziness of the West?

Insomnia culture warps everything it touches.

> I have insomnia all the time, so does my mom. Since I started
> taking my 'smoky brain meds' my insomnia is far less frequent,
> but I also have major OCD, and that keeps me up for hours
> sometimes, because my brain won't let me sleep.
>
> – L, Toronto

Nobody – nobody – is winning the War on Sleep. Unless you count international mega-capital – but corporations are only considered 'persons' in the United States.

Here is what we know: the Twenty-Four-Hour Workday, arguably still more myth than fact in the daily lives of Western citizens (but a myth so strong it makes us behave as if we really do work twenty-four hours a day), exacts a powerful toll, and pull, on the already restless mind; advances in communications technology have distinct drawbacks that we have collectively decided to ignore; profits have never been higher for the commercial institutions that run our society, and we're the ones stuffing the stockholders' pockets.

It's hard to argue with that. You hear such talk every day. You even get angry about it. But it's a casual, scattered sort of anger, not the kind that will make anyone do anything to change the situation. It's a discontent that comes from knowing you have willingly painted yourself into a corner because the colour of the paint was so terribly pretty and felt so smooth and easy on the brush.

But easy corporation- and tech-shaming will get us nowhere. Until we recognize that the fantasy possibilities of the Twenty-Four-Hour Workday are wildly seductive because they speak to our still-lingering modernist urges to live sleeker, more mechanized lives, whisper to us that if only we work more and for longer and longer hours, the same mega-capital riches we now bolster will bolster us. And until we acknowledge that we are as much in love with our sleeplessness, both as a metonym for abundant productivity and as a morbid act of inverse bravado, we will be wide awake until our bodies and the corporate body finally, perhaps irrevocably, collapse.

The image of the ideal worker has radically shifted – no longer the robotic, anonymous drones of Fritz Lang's 1927 film *Metropolis*, today's ideal worker is tasked with being both as productive and undemanding as a drone while also being a well-rounded, creative individual. The ideal worker clocks a forty-hour workweek (which, with added after-office hours, is in reality closer to sixty hours), and then, somehow, magically finds time to hike, do charity work and write a clever blog.

Young people vying for their first jobs are instructed by career counsellors to discuss their 'hobbies' (an antiquated word, given that the off-hours leisure culture that supported the boom in hobby culture in the last century, and the idea of doing an activity purely for whatever rewards it might give, are both dead concepts) and their volunteer work, as well as their larger life goals. Any potential employee who tells the truth, that after work they crawl home, spend too many hours managing all of their online lives and then collapse in a heap, would be read by an interviewer as lazy, self-indulgent and likely morally bankrupt.

This image of a 'full life' (that feeling full can also be as uncomfortable as a stomach ache we will set aside), one wherein the work we do is made better by the activities we pursue when not working, and wherein said activities are nourished by our for-money labours, is a fabrication that neatly fits into the same late-capitalist ideology that presents money and money-chasing not as an end goal, something dirty but necessary, but rather as a breathing, twinkling, pulsating river of life. We are told that only those of us who live parallel to the river of information, who stay in sync with its allegedly fascinating ebb and flow, will ever thrive, or just survive. I believe this myself, despite knowing better.

In a 2007 thesis entitled *Personal Consequences of Work Under 'New Economy,'* prepared for Middle East Technical University's (METU) Graduate School of Social Sciences, C. Metin Kodalak argued, 'Under the "new economy" conditions, employees have to be healthy and dynamic for 7/24. When the economy is dependent upon short-term, any breakdown … should be avoided.' This much was obvious a decade ago, and is decidedly worse now.

What Kodalak notes later, however, is more revealing. When asked if they found such precarious and health-threatening working conditions troublesome, most employees questioned 'prefer those kinds of insecure jobs despite the hardship involved,' because the 'challenge of technology and other employees is preferred.'

In other words, the 'highly-qualified white-collar professionals' interviewed (most of whom worked out of Technopolis, a bustling new industrial-tech park connected to METU's Ankara campus) found the health risks and related vulnerabilities a good trade-off for the excitement of their new occupations. That was 2007. If anything, such occupations are now more seductive than ever, and are hardly restricted anymore to the tech industries, because *everything* is now part of the tech industry.

Kodalak goes on to describe these 'honey trap jobs' as 'promising autonomy and the control of time,' but as actually causing 'employees [to] in fact sink into the heavy load of work and forced to work for more "flexible" hours. As with work-related stress, burn-out is also becoming prevalent under the modern conditions of work. Burn-out, as mentioned here, is characterized with "emotional exhaustion," "de-personalization," "experience of poorer performance" and "cynicism" (Altieri et. al., 2005:158). Burn-out is common especially among managers or young professionals due to intense work.'

'Still, flexible work continues to be used in the advantage of companies,' Kodalak says. 'This one-way time-lengthening flexibility is valid almost for all companies in METU-Technopolis. Moreover, the impossibility of maintaining the heavy tempo of working intensely causes anxiety for the young employees. As an example, an electronic engineer aged twenty-six expresses: "I can work with a high performance for now. I have headaches, backaches, but I can resist. I know I will not show such a performance when I am thirty-five ... [for now] I have to be indispensable for the company, otherwise fear takes over."'

I wonder where that anxious young man is today? He'd be over thirty-five now.

Kodalak concludes the study of the health risks associated with the Twenty-Four-Hour Workday by noting, 'The intensification, high speed and changes in the forms of work reflected the appearance of new types of work-related problems. Eye problems stemming from continuous working in front of computer, musculoskeletal disorders such as backache, neck hernia, and problems related with the spine, wrist and finger articulations, slimming of leg muscles and getting fat and psychological problems such as stress and insomnia are becoming prevalent with the changing work conditions.

'Even though these problems occur due to long hours of stressful work, it is indispensable for METU-Technopolis companies to work for long hours, including all night and weekends when the project deadline is closer. Although these periods are seen as temporary, indeed intensive work rhythm has become normalized and regular. An employee marks that: "If you are in software sector, you have to stand it. This is the part of it."'

Two things strike me after reading this thesis, a study researched and presented almost ten years before I began this book: first, how innocent the alarm-bell-ringing seems, how if I presented this as a new study, even non-academics would shrug it off as a series of obvious assertions; and second, despite the fact that even so-called 'emerging economies' like Turkey's had their own canaries in the coal mine years ago, nothing has changed for the better.

An ugly irony is that many of the sleep-deprived workers described in Kodalak's study would be regarded today as members of the creative class — workers whose fertile imaginations and energetic, timely responses to the prevailing culture are to be mined for profit, cultivated for their innovative impulse. But how can people continue to create month after month, year into year, when their bodies are falling apart and their brains are exhausted? What will a creative class manufacture in a sleepless future?

Unless our simultaneous dependence and dissociation from insomnia culture is subject to a massive overthrow by medical and/or legal interventions, a movement popularizing more self-determined life choices and a revolution in personal habits, we will remain stuck in a pattern of stress/culturally vacant relief/stress, which will tax our collective creativity until the only thing left is a seemingly thriving culture that is in actuality nothing more than the systemic playing out of endless loops of reflexive and counter-reflexive responses.

In the arts, we will run out of situations and actions to modify with 'post-' and likely retreat to an earlier form of cultural sharing based on place of origin or habitation, or perhaps, more darkly, identity. Not that cultures need universally shared experiences — and certainly not agreed-upon tastes — to function peacefully; however, as insomnia culture breeds a more and more intense pursuit of the 'authentic' as a satisfaction replacement for actual mental rest, an increased sense of maddening unreliability, in all pursuits, is inevitable. The 'true' (when defined as something undiscovered by the many or, much more perishable, as being wholly without guile) is by nature an unsustainable resource, while artificiality, in its very unnaturalness, easily self-replicates, is designed to remake and contort. Insomniac culture is as incapable of resting as it is of allowing for or providing rest.

Twenty-Four-Hour Morning
On sleeping with the fishes

I met the Icelandic sleep expert Dr. Karl Karlsson in early January of 2015, in his home city of Reykjavik. Iceland in January is an odd place to visit if you're experiencing sleep difficulties. The sun rises around 10:30 or later in the morning, stays low in the horizon, just under the 45-degree angle, and then slowly, almost reluctantly, begins to sink back under the horizon in a blast of gold, starting around 2:30 p.m. and finally disappearing just before 5. When the sun is up and out, the light is diamond bright and even a bit harsh. Weirdly, the daytime seems rather long, drawn-out. Perhaps it is the angle of the sunlight? The brain reads the day as being one long morning.

Dr. Karlsson teaches and researches at the University of Reykjavik, a small but teeming campus located on the outskirts of the city. U of R is anchored by a new glass, steel and blue-grey stone building that resembles a frozen pond turned upside down. We meet for a chat in the building's centre, where a non-stop stream of young students converges to guzzle coffee and play with their phones. Dr. Karlsson is handsome, in a scruffy sort of fashion, and, like all the men in Iceland, sports a wayward beard. His tattoos betray his years of study and work in the U.S. (most Icelandic academics look more like business people).

Dr. Karlsson began his career studying respiratory health and then became interested in the science of sleep. He completed his PhD at the University of Iowa, specializing in the development and stages of sleep in rats. His post-doctoral studies focused on known neural systems doing unknown neural things, 'behaving strangely,' which led to the further study of the neural connections established in non-normative neurological events. Because rat brains have been so thoroughly studied, the patterns of neural connections, and variants from the norm, are more easily mapped.

Specifically, Dr. Karlsson studied the ontogency of sleep patterns in rats (*ontogency* describes biological patterns charted throughout the whole life of a species). But with brains, rat or human, Dr. Karlsson informs me, there is no strict wiring formula in neurological patterns. 'Imagine,' he suggests, 'the brain as a ball of wires. The development of the brain is the process of stringing those wires together. I am interested in variations in the wiring patterns from "normal" patterns.'

Post-doctoral work in Los Angeles followed, and Dr. Karlsson was part of a team that specialized in studying a single peptide called orexin. Orexin is a chemical that is missing from the brains of people who suffer from narcolepsy. For some little-understood reason, the neurons that produce orexin have died in the brain. Part of the reason Dr. Karlsson returned to Iceland is that, as he puts it, 'the field of neurology, especially in the discovery and study of peptides and other chemicals, is extremely competitive and yet the actual studies are very random, because there is little co-operation between study groups.' In Iceland, he tells me, he can work outside of 'the mad race' of U.S. biochemical research.

'But this is Iceland,' he says, shrugging. 'We don't have the same money and level of research resources. We can get rats in Iceland for science, but no money for anything else, because rats are so expensive. So I use zebra fish, about two thousand of them – if you have an aquarium, you know zebra fish: they are small, black-and-white-striped fish that people like to keep in groups because they school. We use zebra fish because they have nervous systems and spines, and now their genome has been sequenced and their behaviour can be quantified. Zebra fish have not been used much in research, so they are also "low-hanging fruit," so to speak.'

My first question for Dr. Karlsson is an obvious one. 'What are the similarities between sleep in fish and sleep in humans?'

'When we talk about sleep in humans today, we talk almost exclusively about brainwaves. But brainwaves are not always useful as a sole diagnostic tool. With animals, because they do not develop the same way as humans – on any level, but especially the brain – we understand that the definition of sleep actually changes too. This allows us to study other aspects of sleep. Brainwaves are only one way to define sleep. Because of this focus on brainwaves, our definitions of sleep describe what is basically a middle-aged white male phenomenon – because that group is both the funder of and thus the subject of the science.

'Why the focus on brainwaves?' I ask.

'The main reason,' says Dr. Karlsson, 'is that it took a long time to develop a consensus about what sleep actually is – and, this is true, funny as it sounds, that "consensus" was agreed upon at a cigar meeting, an old boys' club meeting, in 1968 or 1969, between the most powerful scientists in the field at the time ... who happened to be middle-aged white men. And then that so-called consensus turned into dogma. It got to the point where EEG, which is just a measurement, became an activity in itself, not a corollary to sleep. Also, the medical industry has profited because this dogma and this consensus make everything faster and standardized. Having an easy standard model for what constitutes sleep makes things very easy for the industry.

'After that consensus became standard, people wanted to start to apply genetic models to sleep, as genetic studies leapt forward, and who knows what we might have learned? But genetic modelling does not work well with EEG. What we need to better understand sleep is not one thing absolutely or another thing absolutely, but combinations of events and biological mapping in co-operation, and this is important, with a behavioural understanding of sleep.

'This is why I work with fish,' Dr. Karlsson explains. 'Think how easy it is to disrupt sleep and to relapse – or not – into sleep … This also works with flies and fish. They also display the same patterns when they are deprived of sleep. This means we can apply behavioural patterns to sleep events and then, with thousands of fish monitored at once, create quantifiable models of that behaviour. Thousands of fish can be studied at once and we can turn the results into numbers. From that, we can test new drugs, do pharmaceutical tests on the fish by applying the various medications and components in the medications, the different chemicals, to the fish and then generate quantifiable results. Each compound of the new medication can be tested and measured.'

An unhappy thought: I'm a middle-aged white man (and so is Dr. Karlsson), and if all the medications and treatments I have been exposed to don't work, despite the entire system using my 'type' as the medical and investigatory 'standard,' then nothing will work for me. I breathe and consider what might be available to me, and everybody else, if the sleep-science community had taken a moment to examine its own biases and attempt to find resolutions to long-standing problems by exploring how non-Western, non-white and middle-aged, non-male sleep disorder sufferers, and, more importantly, the culture around them, deal with sleep problems.

Dr. Karlsson yawns and slurps down some more coffee. He seems tired and yet wide awake, like all the sleep specialists I've met. I needle him a bit. 'Do you practice what doctors call "good sleep hygiene" yourself?'

'No!' he blurts out, as if I've caught him doing something bad. 'I know so much about insomnia and I still break all the rules, all the time. It's stupid of me. I have night terrors as well, but I don't practice what I know. And I will not use pills, because I know I would abuse them. I work fifty to seventy hours a week. A typical day for me is to work until 5 or 6 p.m., go home and watch the news, then read all night or sit up in bed with my laptop. And I work one weekend a month.'

When I tell him I've heard that before, he nods, as if to say, *Of course you have.* 'What do you think of the scare tactics doctors use, such as "insomnia is the new tobacco"? Do they work on you?'

Dr. Karlsson surprises me. 'These tactics are perfectly reasonable, if they work. People *should* be scared. For instance, there was a big study published a few years ago arguing that the cheaper it is to make light, to turn night into day, really, the less people sleep. Before gas lighting, when lights were minimal and expensive for nighttime for most people, there was no activity. People stopped doing things. Now we have colonized the night. And with LEDs becoming better and cheaper and more common – they are 25 per cent cheaper than incandescent light, the pattern or erasing nighttime, and darkness, and being more active at night, will only grow stronger. It will cut one hour, economically speaking, from the already not enough six hours we spend in darkness. Also, LEDs create more blue light, and blue light connects to the eyes and then shuts off melatonin, so the effect cascades forward.

'Maybe there are no more "normal sleep" people, and we should stop thinking about trying to restore any idea of "normal" and instead work on individual sleep health? Because it is impossible to go back to more night. Nobody wants to do that, and the economy would collapse if we did.'

The economy would collapse if we did. Isn't that the response to every proposed overhaul of changes to the way work and health collide? As Kodalak's study from nearly a decade ago demonstrates, not sleeping in order to be productive first starts as a kind of challenge, almost a sport, particularly among young workers. Then it morphs into a practice, a routine, and, because it generates more profits, becomes codified or indirectly codified by management (the worker who sleeps less makes more). After this happens, it's a short jump to normalization: everyone is sleeping less and working more, and to rationalize this, workers begin to see sleep as the enemy of profit. Sleep self-deprivation is, by consensus, the norm — a norm shared by millions to the point that it marks a dramatic cultural shift. When one looks at the overall shift in the perception of sleep's value, one sees it as a kind of accidental plot against the worker — as if employers, noticing that workers are willing to forgo sleep for rewards, institutionalized a system of labour practices that both anticipate and demand that workers sleep less. All the while, everyone knows this unfolding dynamic is doomed to fail, but the up-front rewards are simply too tempting, perhaps even intoxicating over a long period of time, like a sleep-deprivation-generated hallucination played out on a world-wide economic scale. It's like driving toward a destination but staring at the fuel meter hovering over the E, and driving on anyway – an act of both hope and denial only occasionally interrupted by hard second thoughts.

When I suggest that the Icelandic winter, with its miserly dose of sunlight, must be difficult for Icelanders to endure, and must lead to culturally embedded sleep-disruptive behaviours, Dr. Karlsson surprises me again.

'Icelanders have a different language around this time of year and the darkness. We use words like *cozy* to describe the time of year, instead of negative connotation words like *bleak*. We have re-ordered our thinking, over hundreds of years, to embrace the light changes in different times of the year. For instance, Icelanders do not get seasonal affective disorder. Even Icelandic Canadians do not get it! Our culture prioritizes closely knit communities and families — however you define family — and that prevents SAD, because your loved ones are all around you all the time. Think about how people live in other parts of the world — with everybody in their own little rooms, by themselves. I was amazed by that when I first went to the U.S.

'Again, however, the Icelandic reaction to winter, to so-called "light deprivation," is very under-studied. The way Nordic people react to abundant darkness could be a behavioural study that would help people with sleep issues in many ways, but it is not being studied other than as a cultural curiosity. But let's not be sentimental either. Icelanders are like everybody else in the West — we have our devices and toys and lots of artificial light and artificial environments, so maybe in a generation we will not be able to talk about ourselves and our relationship to darkness in the same way.'

So, even a people like the Icelanders, people who have found ways to conquer sleep issues because of their environment and its necessities, might be on the way to naturalizing not-sleeping?

'It is unfortunate, this naturalizing,' Dr. Karlsson admits, 'but I have no idea how to turn back the clock. I have two kids, one is twenty-one and one is fourteen. My kids do things to their sleeping health that would have been unthinkable when I was their age, thirty years ago. My fourteen-year-old would rather lose her arm than her smart phone and my twenty-one-year-old lives all hours, with no two days alike, except that he does not ever sleep enough or properly and is always tired but wide awake. They have no circadian rhythms, none, just like teenagers all over the world now. They are almost like invalids, and I say that because they are exactly like all of their friends, so it is not particular to them.

'We have a whole class now of young people who can't function in the world of nine to five, because they cannot sleep in a regular way, mostly by their own doing. What will happen to them? Will they be dependent on the state? (I mean this larger class, not necessarily my own kids.) We in the West and here in Iceland are normalizing not only sleeplessness but all the lifestyle and social implications of what is essentially a biological disruption. We have made a biological disruption normal, even "cool," and perhaps even something to aspire to. And you cannot separate the social consequences from individual health concerns. We keep talking about insomnia and poor sleep like it is a person-to-person issue, not a social issue.

'For instance,' Dr. Karlsson adds, 'think about not only how we live but in what spaces we live and how we share geographies. If we did not need to sleep, our communities and cities would look completely different. You can eat anywhere, you can clean yourself anywhere – I eat in my office all the time, and the university has showers – but you can't sleep anywhere. You need a specific place and furniture. And sleep dictates how society functions – so if you mess with sleep patterns and sleep health, you are messing with the actual fabric of society. This is a bigger issue than so-and-so the individual patient can't sleep.'

Dr. Karlsson then asks me to think about how much of any community's infrastructure is dictated by the need to sleep – from the direction of roads designed to get commuters back to their beds faster, to the subsequent placement of everything from power generators to water-purification plants. A community starts with a bed. Diminish the role and value of the bed, and its primary purpose – sleep – and you diminish the role and value of community-building itself. Which, perversely, feeds into the repositioning of the ideal worker as a person producing and producing without need of not only sleep, but sleep's many epiphenomena: a sense of home, the creation of safe space that excludes the outside world, the gut need for privacy and comfort and familiarity, for inclusion in the rhythms of nature, the building of a world of one's own, a world that is wholly apart from one's work, a place where one need not be 'on' at all times.

What will the future look like if we don't change?

'We are very close to being able to artificially change our sleep patterns and biological sleep needs,' Dr. Karlsson explains. 'To live with less sleep, but artificially. A change in society will automatically follow. We will loosen the basic agreements and contracts of living together in a society to be more varied, more flexible to the rhythms of people outside of "normal," or what will be called "old-fashioned" sleep habits. There will be classes of people who are richer because they can buy the artificial sleep-changing devices or medicines, and thus work more, and there will be a – probably lower-paid – class of people who will work all night to provide services for the sleepless.

'Maybe this will be more freeing, and that generation I talked about earlier, the young people who can't function nine to five, will have opportunities because the world of business and work will be more flexible – but it will not be a healthier world. And as we experiment with these new arrangements, we are doing it without recognizing that it will take decades and a generation or more to figure out how, or if, this new society of mixed sleepers will even work. But we go forward anyway. In sleep studies, from a sociological perspective, we are basically back in the 1910s.'

Here I disagree with Dr. Karlsson. There is nothing liberating about living without enough sleep or training the body to extend its capacity to stay awake. It is undoubtedly profitable, and yes, a generation trained to constantly rene-gotiate a fundamental need with both their own bodies and their employers might well enjoy a short flourish, a brief era of limitless productivity. But that is not liberation, it's self-enslavement. And once capital convinces a generation of workers to live 'post-sleep,' it will only seek out other core human activities to gradually eradicate, because if one bodily necessity is deemed counter to profit, why not another? Take, for instance, the traditional lunch break. A generation ago, it was an hour. Now the standard is thirty minutes, and many workers eat lunch at their desks, so they can keep up.

Now apply that shrinking of off-duty time to sleep. It's a frightening image.

'All we can do now,' says Dr. Karlsson, 'is monitor patterns as they emerge, and try to deduce what to do, if anything. But there is no way to apply science and tests to this with animals, because, of course, animals don't make themselves stay up all night, so there is a whole field of test modelling that is not available to us. Again, all we can do is study behaviour, and we don't do that enough.'

It occurs to me that of the many people I have spoken to regarding the growth of insomnia culture, Dr. Karlsson, a man who studies the microscopic intricacies of tiny fish brains all day, is the only person who has made the connection between cultural shifts – 'behaviour,' as he puts it – and their consequences.

A side note and coincidence: The same week I met with Dr. Karlsson, the *Reykjavik Grapevine*, a popular Icelandic English-language weekly newspaper, published an interview with Erla Bjornsdottir, a psychologist practicing in the city. Regarding seasonal affective disorder, Bjornsdottir is quoted as saying, 'My feeling as a working psychologist is that SAD rates are high here [in Iceland],' and that 'now is the peak time in my clinic, we have a long waiting list' – in other words, the opposite of Dr. Karlsson's evaluation. Furthermore, Bjornsdottir claims that Icelanders have 'the world record in hypnotics use ... Last year there were eight million sleeping tablets prescribed here [in Iceland], which is crazy [the Icelandic population hovers around a mere 300,000 people]. In some age groups,' Bjorns-dottir remarks, 'we have 70 per cent using sleeping tablets.' Her solution is to change the Icelandic national clock so that 'what little daylight we have [is shifted] to the morning.'

Obviously, Dr. Karlsson and Erla Bjornsdottir have one fundamental disagreement about the prevalence of seasonal affective disorder (and its co-symptom, sleep disruption), but a hybrid of their theories might work. What if Iceland attempted a social experiment that first altered the clock to allow for more daylight but also altered the 'work clock' and mandated that Icelanders have shorter working hours in the dark months, so they could literally sleep away the night? There would be an immediate drop in productivity and commerce, but would that soon be followed by a more developed (and thus richer) and more intense form of productivity, one centred on a shorter but far more effective and less stressful workday? If we have so little problem altering our perception of work time vs. rest time with medications – as that is what sleeping pills do, they rejig your body's sleep time – why not take the next step and radically alter (or, perhaps, return to an age-old version of) the concept of daytime/work time and nighttime/rest time itself?

I sleep fairly well if I ignore the seductive call of demon caffeine after twelve noon. This makes teatime an herbal affair. But if Morpheus and I want to link up later for a little bedroom fun, it has to be like this.

– J, Toronto

Podcasts are my cure for an overly busy nighttime brain. The story distracts from my own crap and the voice lulls me off. Even if I wake up several times, I seem to have trained myself to nod off again after five minutes of *History of the World in 100 Objects*, Melvin Bragg or Ira Glass.

– M, St. John's

I have always had a fragile relationship with sleep … More nights than not I am up in the middle of the night for a couple of hours, angst-ridden about something or another – whatever it is, it all seems pretty silly in the light of day.

– N, Toronto

Sleep is a fragile commodity. Everyone I spoke to during the writing of this book, even friends who have never experienced more than a fleeting episode of insomnia, described their elaborate sleep rituals, rules and the stringent and never-varied-from conditions under which they acquired sleep. We talk about sleep the way farmers talk about growing delicate crops, or birdwatchers talk about spotting rare species. Even the well-slept are anxious about their sleep, the continuation of their good run.

All this trepidation betrays a compensatory impulse, a feeling that if one does not guard against sleep interruption, sleep will not come – an impulse that, conscious or not, further betrays a larger cultural anxiety over sleep in general. Without sleep, the entire, allegedly life-defining project of making and profiting collapses, but everyone who makes and profits is also now expected to be awake longer, in order, of course, to make more and (allegedly) profit more. This formula is not sustainable. Everyone knows it is not sustainable, even people who never worry about sleep personally, because they are surrounded by the sleep-deprival worries of their friends, lovers and co-workers and because insomnia culture's signifiers remind us constantly that we live in a world where being under-slept is naturalized and often vaunted.

A collision is inevitable, a collision between the multiple forces that disable sleep, from profit-chasing to cultural mass dissociation, and the inescapable needs of the human body. How will this collision and the aftershock play out? I can only predict a dystopian future, one populated by two types of worker-citizens: those who have found a way around sleep needs, or have resigned themselves to living shorter but highly profitable lives; and the less fortunate, who will be read as a drag on society at best and live horribly marginalized existences at worst. Only from this point of absolutes and extremities will real change emerge. Until then, it's a game of catch-up, ever increasing in speed and relentlessness.

4 a.m. The early morning prompts stupid romanticisms. Sunrise, the first birds, cats on the make, rough garbage collectors and howling drunks, the lazier sorts of ghosts. All true, the first thirty or so times, all perversely exciting, edgy and uncanny. The world simply looks different in the morning – less defined and thus less exacting. The first few dozen times.

How it turns.

Daybreak mists, once so fresh and moist, grow mildew, sit in the lungs like wet flour. The imprecise corners of buildings, so charmingly velveteen the first time around, now menace and appear unstable. Those birds are not singing, they're begging, squawking against the sun, the new, dangerous day, against the light that wakes every other creature, every damned animal that hunts and eats.

The sweet routine of morning chores and morning tasks unveils itself, at last, shows what it really is – a grind, a mandatory expenditure of energy for expenditure's sake. Storefronts are swept with a grunt, not a whistle. Your neighbour stands in his kitchen, the ends of his tie dangling from around his neck, gulping coffee and rubbing his burning stomach. The pretty, shiny new morning is suddenly exposed for what it really is: grubby, rushed and deprived, a world clotted with the night's grime, that crusty gunk that clogs the corners of your waking eyes, shaken awake by a hacking cough.

So much for romance. I once dated another insomniac. He was great fun everywhere but in bed (we often had sex on the floor, on a chair – never his bed). He told me once that after years of not sleeping, he had grown to loathe his bed, the actual square of mattress he crawled into every night. He called it his 'torture mat.' He didn't like to sit on it, let alone fool around on it.

And yet he couldn't live without a bedroom and a mattress because someday that traumatized space might fulfil its promises, might provide sleep and rest, so why take the chance? One night we were listening to music and I casually asked him what his favourite sounds were. 'I know what I hate,' he said. 'I hate the sound of birds.' Birds, he told me, reminded him of how he had failed, again, to sleep. Birdsong always sounded like cruel laughter to him, jeers. When he heard the morning birds chattering, he got out of bed and gave up, resigned himself to another night of losing the sleep game. Birds were on the 'other team,' nature's team, and he was outside of nature, a failed animal. No wonder he didn't want to fuck in bed – imagine the pressure.

People who are awake just before dawn and not out having fun are a miserable people. We consider the day ahead of us and wonder how we can make it to the long, far-away end. We wonder why we are cursed. We fantasize about every sort of knockout scenario: suicide (which, granted, sounds romantic in the Goethe sense of the word, but is really rather low-rent and churlish, without sweeping gestures or thunderous finales); monkish retreats into remote, underpopulated lands (I once spent the dead hours thoroughly investigating how to acquire residency in Bhutan); simply giving up and staying in bed forever, letting go of the idea of ever being a part of the larger world.

People who are awake before dawn but don't want to be are natural dramatists, 'scripters' in the language of cognitive disorder studies. We think we can see the future (and, in a way, therefore can). We convince ourselves our hated apartness gives us the gifts of extra sight, extra perception and magical powers (again, of the low-rent, sympathetic magic variety, which is often little more than simple herbalism, spice-drawer aromatherapy, hot baths and minted hot milk).

When you are deprived of a basic life function, and have tried all the 'real' remedies, magic is never far off in your mind. The world is full of witch doctors, a description I consider complimentary and worthy, for a reason.

Insomniacs also learn that we are not alone. It takes only a handful of up-all-night nights to figure out who else is up all night. Televisions give people away, and computer screens, all the blue and white lights that pulse and jump behind curtains.

I can't be the only insomniac who has looked out his living room window and thought, *Why don't we all get together? We're awake. We could swap sleep recipes, console each other, plot terrible crimes.* But it won't happen, any gathering of the near-dead, because the only thing more abhorrent to a restless mind in the ugly hours than the actual harshness of the ugly hours is the thought of having to listen to somebody else. Somebody else in distress, also angry at the comfortable world.

Whenever someone tells me, in an attempt to bond with my chronic insomnia, that they too are, at heart, a 'night person,' I nod and listen and think, *Be careful what you ask for*, because of course true 'night people' want nothing more than to never face another long, aimless, frustrating night again. We want perpetual sun. We want the world to be reset in our key, to our broken rhythm. We want the world turned upside down.

Funny how everyone I've ever met who describes himself or herself as a night person looks perfectly well-rested, full-blooded and luminous.

Amateurs.

Restless leg syndrome continues to frustrate my attempts to live a healthier life (granted, 'healthy' is a culturally loaded concept, but we'll let that slide). One evening, after spending all day writing about RLS, I was chatting with an old friend about RLS and my attempts to accurately convey how the syndrome plays out in my body when, out of nowhere (nowhere, because she sleeps like an angel), my pal suggested that I take a mystical approach to the situation (I am a bit of a witch).

Perhaps, she proposed, your legs, and the rest of twitching you, act out such violent agitations because your spirit knows that should you go to sleep, darker, more malevolent forces will take over your mind in the form of nightmares and visions? Your body is protecting you from, essentially, the demonic, she argued. Better awake and flailing than asleep and terrorized.

To an outsider, the above sounds lunatic, or at least very west coast, like something of and for the fairies. But I am, first off, no stranger to occultist beliefs, and, more important, her idea caused me to remember one terrible night when I was about twelve. For reasons I no longer remember, I became convinced I was possessed by Satan, in body and spirit. Sometime well past midnight, I lay awake in a state of pure terror while a coinciding (or symptomatic of demonic possession?), ferocious attack of RLS caused me to crack and then dislodge the cheap pine headboard at the top of my bed.

My parents heard the crash and came into my room. I have a vivid memory of looking up at both of them – my father on the left, my mother on the right – as they stood over me and tried to shake me awake (but of course I was already awake: I was having a fit).

My mother asked me, each time in a louder and more alarmed voice, what was wrong, what was wrong, what was wrong? I could not speak, and I could not stop thrashing around the bed. I remember whispered talk about 'the outdoor' (a New Brunswick term for an emergency room), and hearing my father tell my mother to slap me, for my own good. I may have wet myself, but I am not certain if that is just me trying to add literary value to the story. I do remember, with bald certainty, my mother trying to hold me down and my father wondering aloud if I was 'faking' (he was not a good parent).

And then, the attack – demonic or just hysteric – stopped. My legs flattened on the bed; I was lucid. 'I had a nightmare,' I said, and that was enough to prompt my father to leave with a few choice curse words and his usual observation that he regretted having a second child. My mother stayed with me until I fell asleep.

Maybe, as happened way back then, my RLS and the disorder's damned attendant metaphors will shut off again, just like that, for reasons I will never know (nor truly care to find out about)? Maybe this long battle will just stop, will end as capriciously as it currently flares up, become utterly tired of torturing me and move on to some other hapless body?

Maybe the demons will float away, find viler bodies to overrun. Maybe, one night, I will kick myself free.

Self-improvement guru Dale Carnegie once said, 'If you can't sleep, then get up and do something important instead of lying there worrying.' The 'important' in that sentence cuts deepest. Carnegie believed in, and successfully sold, the idea that all human problems could be overcome with positive thinking and hard work. It's easy to be cynical about his philosophy, but there is no denying the potency of his world view, how much it still influences how we think about our health.

Can't sleep? Well, you've just got too much time on your hands and not enough to do with those idle paws. Every insomniac believes this to be true, as neurotics are very good at self- blame. We believe that ultimately our health is a problem of our own making – that, and many other unpleasant narratives. What have I done with all those thousands of hours spent in bed, fretting? So little, and nothing Carnegie-esque. I could have written ten more books, made hundreds of new friends, met a lover, found a cure – done anything but worry about the fact that I was not asleep.

Insomniacs are not good at forgiveness. We are natural grudge holders, as are most people out of sync with nature. So, for us to forgive ourselves for being chronically awake … what was Dr. Dang-Vu's phrase, for having poor 'sleep hygiene'? (a term I love for its clinical resonance and the way it makes sleeplessness seem so manageable, like keeping up with one's laundry) … well, that's more or less the same as asking us to simply fix ourselves, which would include, first and paradoxically, forgiving ourselves.

I cannot, not yet. I'm afraid that if I set aside my rage and frustration, I will never find a fix for my inability to sleep – and I'm keenly aware at the same time that rage and frustration keep me up at night. Perhaps insomnia is just displaced fury, an internalized lashing out?

When I started writing this book, I expected to end it with definite answers. I dreamed of a cure, one that I would uncover like a detective or investigative journalist, a cure not *only* for myself, but, to be blunt, *mostly* for myself. No two insomnias are alike, after all.

I thought I could write a normal sleeping life into existence, make regular and restful sleep 'manifest,' as occultists call the making of one thing from another but intangible thing, and create a new relationship between myself and the old mattress. And then, from that momentous shift, I would gain a new body, a new outlook, a less fraught life. Instead, I learned rather a lot of alarming things and a handful of hopeful ones too. I have tried to be reasonable.

I take no solace in the fact that Western culture is moving toward an acceptance of insomnia as part of the cost of contemporary life, or at least a successful contemporary life. A world full of people like me is terrifying to me, and ought to be terrifying to you, as it will not be an easygoing, frolicsome world. A world run by insomniacs will be a resigned world, one with little energy to confront challenges and zero desire to be or create anything that is more than mildly stimulating. Such a world will also be, perversely, a comfort-geared world, one overstuffed with soft textiles and twinkling, subliminally nod-along- (but never dance-) worthy music, a world of bubble baths and clean, fresh scents. A dull hell.

The few sleepers left, if for no reason better than resentment of the fluffy and undemanding world around them, will morph into something akin to first-wave punks. Theirs will be a world of noise and grime, their lives ones of solitude interrupted by the occasional company of the fellow disgruntled. How they will hate our fleecy, sober world. Given that people who sleep less and less will be rewarded for their (albeit short-term) faux but instantly gratifying (to their bosses) productivity, a sneering resentment of the insomniac's padded, boring, nap-time world could come, of all places, from the born wealthy, not the employed classes.

The rich will cultivate shock and stimulation, the rest of us predictability and numbing. The well-off, and thus well-slept, will live lives crammed with novelty, as they did in every other era before the modern, but with an especial twist – they will crave discomfort, because all around them the culture will offer products and services and entertainments devised to soothe.

Another possible scenario is that in half a generation everyone, from every class, will be doped up to the gills, highly dysfunctional and on the verge of physical collapse. Sudden breaks from reality will be the norm, and we will teach ourselves to work around mental disruptions, our own and those displayed by others. Our concept of what is 'crazy' and what is not will be very fluid and casual, because none of us will be far from our own breakdowns (which we will be expected to medicate ourselves out of in a matter of minutes).

In either scenario, the sellers of short-term solutions win. They always have.

Acknowledgements

Thanks very much to Jason McBride for encouraging me to write this book, and then to Heidi Waechtler and Alana Wilcox for putting up with me while I wrote this book.

Thanks to my vast collection of attentive and clever friends: Jared Mitchell, Keith Cole, Peter Dube, Dayna McLeod, Suzy McCluskey, Andrew Harwood, Rollin Leonard, Lisa Pereira, Melony Ward, Clarissa Hurley, Robert Windrum, Ken Moffatt, Nora Underwood, all the people who answered my online insomnia quiz, and, especially for his enthusiastic response to my ideas, the always gentlemanly Mr. James R. Tennyson.

Fiona Smyth, you are a joy to work with, now and always.

Thank you to Drs. Chee, Dang-Vu, Karlsson and Little Elk, and my reliable GP Dr. Luetkehoelter.

This book is dedicated to the memory of my mother, Dorothy Frances Vaughan.

About the Author

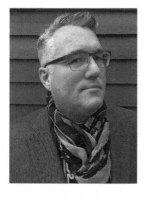

RM Vaughan is a writer and video artist who is originally from New Brunswick and currently lives in Berlin and Toronto.

Vaughan's critically acclaimed books include the poetry collections *A Selection of Dazzling Scarves, Invisible to Predators, Ruined Stars* and *Troubled: A Memoir in Poems and Fragments* (Coach House, 2008), the novels *A Quilted Heart* and *Spells*, the plays *Camera, Woman* (Coach House, 1998) and *The Monster Trilogy* (Coach House, 2003) and *Compared to Hitler: Selected Essays*. Vaughan's essays, poems, fiction and plays appear in over sixty Canadian and international anthologies. Vaughan contributes art criticism and commentary on contemporary culture to numerous publications, and his work has been nominated for the National Magazine Award, the William Kilbourn Award and the ReLit Award.

Vaughan's short videos and video collaborations/installations/performances have played in galleries and festivals around the world.

Works Cited

Jenny Chapman, 'Cambridge Company Mundipharma Gets Approval for Restless Leg Treatment,' Cambridge–News.co.uk, January 8, 2015.

Conversation with Dr. Chee, Toronto Sleep Institute, November 2014, Montreal.

Jonathan Crary. *24/7: Late Capitalism and the Ends of Sleep* (Verso/New Left Books, 2013).

Michael J. Green, Colin A. Espie, Michaela Benzeval. 'The Longitudinal Course of Insomnia Symptoms: Inequalities by Sex and Occupational Class Among Two Different Age Cohorts Followed for 20 Years in the West of Scotland,' *Sleep* (www.journalsleep.org), June 1, 2012.

John F. Kasson. *Houdini, Tarzan and the Perfect Man: The White Male Body and the Challenge of Modernity in America* (Hill and Wang, 2001).

C. Metin Kodalak. *Personal Consequences of Work Under 'New Economy': The Case of METU-Technopolis.* Thesis submitted to the Graduate School of Social Sciences of Middle East Technical University, September 2007.

Lynn Lamberg. 'Insomnia Shows Strong Link to Psychiatric Disorders,' about study by the U.S.-based Institute of Medicine, in Psychiatric News: http://psychnews.psychiatryonline.org/doi/full/10.1176/pn.40.12.00400021

Jonathon Sturgeon. '2014: The Death of the Postmodern Novel and the Rise of Autofiction,' Flavorwire (online), Dec 31, 2014.

Eluned Summers-Bremner. *Insomnia: A Cultural History* (Reaktion Books, 2008).

'Targin Receives Positive European Commission Decision for RLS,' SleepReviewMag.com, January 7, 2015.

'Why Is Everyone So Busy?' *The Economist*, December 20, 2014.

About the
Exploded Views Series

Exploded Views is a series of probing, provocative essays that offer surprising perspectives on the most intriguing cultural issues and figures of our day. Longer than a typical magazine article but shorter than a full-length book, these are punchy salvos written by some of North America's most lyrical journalists and critics. Spanning a variety of forms and genres – history, biography, polemic, commentary – and published simultaneously in all digital formats and handsome, collectible print editions, this is literary reportage that at once investigates, illuminates and intervenes.

www.chbooks.com/explodedviews

Typeset in Goodchild Pro and Gibson Pro. Goodchild was designed by Nick Shinn in 2002 at his ShinnType foundry in Orangeville, Ontario. Shinn's design takes its inspiration from French printer Nicholas Jenson who, at the height of the Renaissance in Venice, used the basic Carolingian minuscule calligraphic hand and classic roman inscriptional capitals to arrive at a typeface that produced a clear and even texture that most literate Europeans could read. Shinn's design captures the calligraphic feel of Jensen's early types in a more refined digital format. Gibson was designed by Rod McDonald in honour of John Gibson FGDC (1928–2011), Rod's long-time friend and one of the founders of the Society of Graphic Designers of Canada. It was McDonald's intention to design a solid, contemporary and affordable sans serif face.

Printed at the old Coach House on bpNichol Lane in Toronto, Ontario, on Rolland Opaque Natural paper, which was manufactured, acid-free, in Saint-Jérôme, Quebec, from 50 percent recycled paper, and it was printed with vegetable-based ink on a 1965 Heidelberg KORD offset litho press. Its pages were folded on a Baumfolder, gathered by hand, bound on a Sulby Auto-Minabinda and trimmed on a Polar single-knife cutter.

Series editor: Jason McBride
Copy edited by Stuart Ross
Series cover design by Ingrid Paulson
Cover illustration by Fiona Smyth (fiona-smyth.blogspot.com)
Author photo by Ryan Vaughan

Coach House Books
80 bpNichol Lane
Toronto ON M5S 3J4
Canada

416 979 2217
800 367 6360

mail@chbooks.com
www.chbooks.com